CW00449961

REIKI

IS

LOVE

Gaetano Vivo

Cover Design, Text and Illustrations copyright © 2007 Gaetano Vivo

First edition published in the United States in 2006 by BookSurge
ISBN 1-4196-2262-5

This second edition published in Great Britain in 2007 by Four O' Clock Press
ISBN13 978-1-906146-21-4

The right of Gaetano Vivo to be identified as the Author of the Work
has been asserted by him in accordance with the Copyright, Designs and
Patent Act 1988

All rights reserved.
No part of this publication may be reproduced, stored in a retrieval system,
or transmitted, in any form or by any means without the prior written
permission of the Author

Printed in the UK by BookForce

Available from Discovered Authors Online –
All major online retailers and available to order through all UK bookshops

Or contact:

Books
Discovered Authors
50 Albemarle Street, London
W1S 4BD
+(44) 207 529 37 29
books@discoveredauthors.co.uk

BookForce UK's policy is to use papers that are natural, renewable and
recyclable products and made from wood grown in sustainable forests
where ever possible

BookForce UK Ltd.
50 Albemarle Street
London W1S 4BD
www.bookforce.co.uk

To my mum forever

TABLE OF CONTENTS

ACKNOWLEDGMENTS

I have received help from many people during the long months of writing this book. First, I want to thank my parents, who have been my Guardian Angels since the moment I was born, for all the love, support, and trust that they have given me. My mom is now watching me from Heaven where she continues to be my Guardian Angel and teacher. My dad, a doctor who is with me in the physical realm, has been a good support throughout my life. Despite his scientific scepticism and good-natured bewilderment at my devotion to what he considers a quixotic pursuit, he continues to love and sustain me in my vocation.

An Angelic thank you to my Spiritual father, mentor and Guardian Archangel Michael, who is there for me everyday of my life, guiding and protecting me and whispering loving thoughts in my mind.

I extend a thank you, also, to my family especially to Gabriella, Ettore, and Vincenzo for their love; and to Flavia, my niece, who is the light of our lives today.

I thank all my friends. I thank, in a special way, for their love and support always: Vincenzo Di Benedetto, Gabriella and Ettore Vivo, Silvana Papa, Nello Cicenia, Giovanna Russo, Anna Paturzo, Gabriella Galgani, Claudia Di Leva, MariaGrazia Panizza, Eleni Scondra, Doreen Wells, Sabrina Del Prete, Jasmine Danda, Lorraine Recchia, Howard Roberts, (my angel friend on Earth), and Tea, the organizer of my seminars in the Canary Islands. .

A great thank you goes to Lisa, my inspirational friend, whose strength and love enabled me to live in America for a while and meet many new friends. Lisa, you are now with the angels. I love you forever. To Kim, who has lost her battle with cancer. I will cherish the deep moments we have spent together forever.

Another special thank you goes to my dear friend Averil Hoole, for all her advice, suggestions, and moral support throughout our many years of friendship and trust.

A big thank you goes to all the artists involved in this project, especially Roberta Collier Morales for her beautiful chakra and symbol illustrations, Armando Pirozzi, for the lovely psychological illustrations and Tony Greco for the special book cover. A special thank you also goes to my dearest friend, Antonella Russo, for modeling and Dino Criscuolo for the photographs. A big thank you goes to Nick Ashron for the picture of Archangel Michael on the back cover.

My health and body were maintained in good shape thank to personal trainer, Terry Rodham, who has allowed my mind to work under good vibes whilst writing this book. I am also grateful to Jo Sensini PR in London and her team for their representation and media advice.

I am most grateful to my teachers; especially to Mr. Arthur Molinary (The Medium) in London, for having helped me, taught me, and inspired me at the beginning of my spiritual development; my Reiki Master Teachers, Shalinda and William Lee Rand, for their teachings; Doreen Virtue PhD, for having shown me the way to the Angelic Realms, Sally Pullinger in Glastonbury through the teachings of the old Chinese have inspired my work even more.

I thank my students all over the world, in USA, Australia, England, Denmark, Norway, Greece, Spain and Italy, for their love and support and for having chosen me as their Reiki Master Teacher.

Finally, I extend my gratitude to the people who have participated with their stories; I continue to be inspired by them.

Disclaimer:

Reiki is not a substitute for any form of medicine or drugs that have been prescribed by practitioners of medicine. In the case of any health emergency, clients should consult their own physicians.

Forward

Reiki is only love. This simple and easy to ready book is a collection of daily stories of women and men who have had the nerve to expose themselves in order to show others the simplicity, joy, and courage it takes to heal oneself. Discover a new approach on how you see Reiki today.

Only with a journey inside, can we appreciate the love that comes from within, doing that, we will be able to help others. This book is yet another book on Reiki but it is also a book of life's affirmations to love; the biggest and greatest love that each one of us desires. We need to feel a sense of brotherhood, a sense of mutual love for one another. The planetary changes we are experiencing, will allow us to fight, to go forward, achieve and love our brothers and sisters all over the world.

If we cannot find peace inside, in our families, peace with friends and relatives, how can we preach peace, how can we give peace.

Turn around, look who is behind you, give them a smile, a hug, do not expect anything in return, this is the best gift of all. Give respect to another being, give them your hand, give them love, and send them love. Always smile, to your children, to your parents, and to strangers. Never be afraid of giving your love to others.

We are all one. When we send love energy, prayers, and loving thoughts to others, this is the best help we can send to the ones in need. It has already happened that with large praying groups, people and places have been healed at a faster pace. Money and commodities are not always the answers to solve problems of starvation, peace, or brotherhood in the world. We need to pray more, to think positively, sending unconditional loving energy to people everywhere.

The power of love is real, the power of love is great. We have been struggling and now we will triumph. There will be a great new Earth for our children to live on. We will be ready when Earth's energy is shifted to be more natural, organic and more earthly.

Everything is happening now. We are ready to shift into the fifth dimension where Earth will be a place of love, joy, and brotherhood. You can see the changes that planet Earth is going through; Volcanoes that explode, Hurricanes and Tornados that destroy everything and kill many, changing seasons, and much more. There will be more, until we learn the way to LOVE.

Introduction

This book is divided in two parts. The first one, is a collection of stories of every day lives. Some were written by me. In the years spent in London, Paris, New York, Boulder, Milan and Naples, I have treated hundreds of people with Reiki and unconditional, angelic, loving energy. Other stories were written by my students, who have had the courage to expose themselves by talking about their own personal development and transformation through Reiki. I think that writing case studies will help people to better understand what Reiki really is in the world today.

Months ago, I asked some of my students to participate in this book with their own stories of how Reiki has transformed their lives and keeps helping them daily. I asked them to only talk about Reiki, and never mention my name; after all, I did not want to bore the reader with the compliments of my students. Ego is not part of my spiritual journey.

The majority of the people though, have thanked me in a way or another. In reading their beautiful stories, I discovered that my name appeared too many times so I have changed a few parts, and for this I apologize to my students and clients.

It is most important that people get benefit from the story they are reading rather then reading about a Reiki Master who has embraced his mission in life to help others to understand.

To all of them this book is dedicated.

All names and places have been changed for privacy.

"I am only a pencil in the hands of God, but it is Him, Him who writes"

Mother Theresa

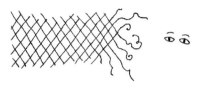

CAROLINA

CAROLINA

A few summers ago, I met Carolina. She was an Italian student who had come to London to learn English. During the summer, I had many visitors staying at my house. That year Carolina was a guest in my house, she was very shy and her parents had preferred her to stay with an Italian person rather that an English family. She was going to stay for three weeks.

One morning, Carolina and I were having breakfast; I could see that her very deep black eyes were desperately trying to tell me something.

Many times people have told me that just being with me put them in a very relaxed peace of mind. Carolina that morning told me that

I

she had suddenly become very curious about my treatments and she wanted to try one.

Carolina was 20; she was very reserved and deep down troubled in some way. She had acne that was spoiling her beautiful little face and because of that, she was afraid of approaching boys.

I did not promise her anything. I told her that we could start a series of therapies and see how we were progressing. I told her that Reiki sometime helps with Self-esteem problems and I felt that her acne was something that was coming from her lack of confidence.

We started the therapies. Carolina was very relaxed and some how I could feel that she trusted my therapy and me completely.

She was very receptive, I remember her sinking, literally, into the treatment table each time she received a treatment and every single time she would go to sleep. When I would wake her up at the end of the treatment, she would come up with incredible stories and vivid dreams that she had gone through during Reiki.

After some treatments, I could see Carolina becoming stronger and happier.

Three weeks passed and time came for Carolina to go back to Milan.

She had become very attached, and I promised her that we would stay in touch.

A few weeks after she left, I received a phone call from Carolina's parents, telling me about her awakening to life. Her mother especially was very pleased by the results; she could see that her daughter had gone through some kind of deep transformation.

A couple of months later, I received a letter from Carolina, telling me that she had finally found the courage to go out with a boy and that she was happy with him, and because of that, her acne was slowing disappearing. She thanked me deeply; she knew that Reiki had helped her more than anything else had before.

I always try to explain to my clients, who tend to put me on a pedestal that it is not me at all. I am only a human being, an ordinary person really, who channels the energy of Reiki that comes through him.

When I teach Reiki classes, I always tell my students to expect this energy going through them. The energy that comes through clears and cleans the energy of the therapist first, and then it is able to flow through the hands of the healer, immaculate and pure.

Carolina is now a happy woman who is accomplishing her Ph.D., and soon will marry her beloved boyfriend.

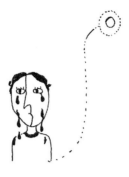

ANTONIO

ANTONIO

Antonio, a young Spanish man, came to see me some time ago. He had never had a Reiki treatment before and hoped that I could heal the skin problems he had suffered for a long time. They had caused him both physical and psychological pains. As I began working on Antonio, I felt some dysfunction in his major chakras, and as I started doing the clearing chakra exercises, all sorts of issues came up for him. Although I had many years of experience in the healing field, I had never seen so much pain coming from a particular individual. While performing the clearing exercise, I could feel Antonio's body almost levitating from the table. It felt like his body had retained a great deal of unwanted energy for a very long time, and through Reiki, the blocked energies could be released.

After four Reiki Treatments, Antonio experienced relief and contentment. He said he felt as if his chakras had been chained for many years and now they felt free, as if they were spinning again. Antonio began to experience positive emotions that he had not felt in a very long time; old issues, some of which he had been unaware, had been cleared forever, leaving him a sense of joy and harmony all over.

Antonio's experience supports the theory that a sane mind allows the body to heal itself.

His mind and body were now healed, and he could proceed on his spiritual journey. Later, I had the honor of training Antonio in the practice of Reiki, and he is now a compassionate and loving Reiki Master.

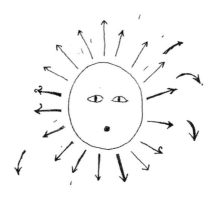

FRANCOISE

FRANCOISE

Francoise was a petite French young woman and a single mum, who would desperately look to use her healing abilities in the best way she could. She came to try a Reiki treatment once, and she remained fascinated by the great energy that would flow through her body.

She had many disappointments in life. She left France at an early age to live and work in England, where she would become a full time nanny. The English adore the fact that their children learn French at an early age.

She had gone through a dysfunctional family and now an abusive husband that she finally decided to get rid of.
Francoise was apparently healthy, with a very strong will. The Reiki

energy worked on her beautifully and each time she would come to receive a treatment her body would absorb all of the energy that it possibly could to make it through for another week.

Francoise became very interested in the Universal Life Energy, to a point where she wanted to learn Reiki. I promised her that she would learn it as soon as she felt better.

She was suffering from something that I could not put my finger on. One evening while I was writing my notes about her, something clicked in my mind. She was possessed by unwanted energies stuck inside her body, and because of that, she could not go forward in life. I had to do something to help her.

I called Francoise and we made an appointment for the next morning. At the same time, I also called two of my Reiki III students to assist me in this process. Maria and Genevieve were two women whom I was training for the Reiki III course of apprenticeship and mastership, which lasts a few years.

They came early that morning. I explained what was going on and that they should keep this matter in confidence. I knew them well enough to trust them on this matter.

We prayed. We cleared the room with the Reiki symbols and we called upon the Energy to assist us in the difficult operation that we were about to start.

Francoise rang the doorbell. She was a bit worried about me calling her but then I explained to her what I thought she was suffering from and she nodded as if she knew exactly what I was talking about.

She agreed that she wanted to go back to her self. Francoise told us that she was ready, she had made a commitment and a promise and she wanted to get rid of the energy that had been bothering her for so many years. She was ready to change and become a successful woman in her own right.

She lay on the treatment table and Maria, Genevieve, and I set out intentions to help her healing.

She was nervous and scared. We were calm and relaxed, knowing that once we came out of this, she would be a new person.

She was now comfortably relaxed on the treatment table and I was seated behind her, touching her shoulders with my hands. Maria and Genevieve were respectively at the left and right of her body. All of a sudden, a strong vibration came and shook her unwanted energy. She started sweating and getting cold. I took a blanket to cover her and she asked me for a second blanket and then a third. She told me that she was freezing and that she did not know whether she could cope with it. We tried to reassure her that everything was fine and the quicker we took away that energy the faster she would heal.

I never call the energy negative energy, is always unwanted, it is energy that the body no longer needs and we are ready to expel it.

As we were giving her Reiki, I felt her body convulsing. She was shaking and scared and I reassured her many times.

All of a sudden, she started screaming like a possessed woman. I had never experienced anything like that. She said that she felt like she was pregnant. With her legs wide open she asked me for a basin,

which Maria promptly got hold of and Francoise started vomiting in. She said, "I am going to give birth, get me some towels!"
I knew she was not pregnant. I prayed for that energy to abandon her body and leave her in peace forever.
We could feel the whole of her body shaking and pulsating, that energy did not want to go; of course, it had been there for so long that it was living in Francoise' body as a parasite.

After much screaming, shouting, and swearing, this energy finally left her body. It was a relief for her. I could see her real face now. She had suffered for many years and her face had turned into a mask of shame, fear, and negativity.

She had returned to the beautiful French flower that she once was. She felt relaxed and happy and had the most beautiful smile I had ever seen on her face.

My two diligent students thanked me for having allowed them to be there with me. They were sure that would help them in their own practice in the future.

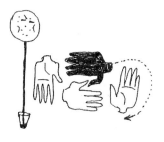

SERENA

SERENA

Serena was a stunning Italian woman from Brooklyn, who had come to follow one of my courses. She was a massage therapist.
She had small but very strong hands that made her massages stronger and deeper. She said that she had seen one of the advertisements about my Reiki courses and she felt interested in following the course from a real Italian.

I noticed Serena's energy as she moved into my space. I could feel a very beautiful loving energy although I knew all along that there was something strange in her.

I always start by balancing the chakras of my students before I start attuning them into the Reiki energy. Each one of my students would be able to tell you exactly how to balance and clear chakras. In turn, I ask my students to be on the treatment table and with the aid of a pendulum I show them how the chakras work and rotate and what to do when the pendulum does not move and why.

It was Serena's turn on the table, she started shaking badly, there was a large unbalance of energy in her body that did not allow her to get any better. Being a massage therapist, she had learned to give excellent and healthy massages but she had never learned how to get rid of people's energy. I thought to my self: *this woman is a sponge, she absorbs unwanted energies from all of her clients and she does not know how to eliminate them.*

Serena was a very good student; she was ready to learn Reiki, even if she had some serious problems. In time she would resolve them.

When a Reiki treatment is performed we enter the aura of the person we are treating at that time. When the treatment is over we are able, with a physical step back, to exit the aura of the person so that all the vibrations stay with the person and do not attack us in any way.

Needless to say, Serena healed in a very short time, after the attunements to Reiki.

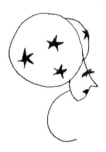

SIGNORA SMITH

THE BARONESS

The baroness was a very wealthy and aristocratic noblewoman from Italy. She was ninety.

She had seen an article about me in an English health publication and she thought I could help her with her sight and lack of memory.

I was used to aristocracy, having lived in England, and I was not surprised, when one morning I got a phone call from a very distinct person who wanted to book an appointment for the baroness.

The morning of the appointment the Lady came to my office in London accompanied by Sonia, her daughter.

They introduced themselves with this very strong accent, and I promptly asked them to speak in Italian.

The baroness was a very frail woman but still very elegant and stylish in her ways. She walked with the aid of two walking sticks, making little steps at the time.

She told me that she was not well, she could no longer see very well and that she was loosing her memory. I thought to myself, *what a beautiful woman, she is more than ninety and still wants to get better and ride the world.* I could see from her face that she had been suffering a lot and working a lot to keep that status of grace that she still had.

She slowly got on the treatment table with my help and her daughter, and I started working on her.

She was grateful. I could feel waves of energy coming, and they would stop at her eyes and her brain.

The head area was where I was treating her; for the memory and the nervous system together with her eye problems. Although during a Reiki treatment you are supposed to stay in position a maximum of three minutes I would work on the baroness far longer.

The baroness came back to me many times as she appreciated my work.
Each time she would tell me how much better she felt, and what an improvement she had found from the previous time. Her daughter was amazed by the results of Reiki and said that she could see symptoms of improvement in her mother's health too.

As the Reiki energy flowed freely in the Baroness's body, her memory began coming back and her sight improved.

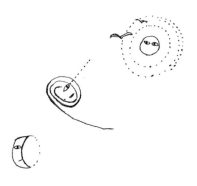

MICHAel

MICHAEL

Michael was a 31-year-old man who loved traveling and experiencing new cultures and new places. He loved to do all the things that people of his age love to do.
He had his whole life ahead of him.

One of his deepest passions was scuba diving. He had many diplomas in this sport; he usually took a scuba-diving trip once a year, somewhere in the world.

One year he decided to go to Florida, to receive a diploma to teach scuba diving. He was happy, because he could from then on teach and be in the water all the time. One very hot day, he decided to take a swim in the hotel pool where he was staying. When he jumped in, he hit his head on the floor of the pool and become unconscious. He woke up in the hospital, completely paralyzed.

His life became turmoil of angry emotions. He returned home, to begin his new life in a wheelchair, requiring a helper to be with him day and night.

One day, I received an E-mail from Michael. He had read an article about Reiki, and was now reading a book about it. He wanted to try it as a new therapy. He had been very interested in other complimentary therapies and he wanted to try Reiki also.

I started seeing Michael once a week at his house.
One day, I asked him if I could bring a group of my Reiki Master trainees with me. He agreed. Going to see Michael, once a week, was a joy for all of us.

Michael eventually asked me to be trained in Reiki. In that way he could give Reiki to himself daily. So it was. Training Michael was one of the most touching experience of my life. It is something that I will cherish forever.

The experience I had with him has been one of growth, for my students as well as me. Michael, of course, is still in the wheelchair but I would like to think that he is happier. He is writing a book on his experience and the effects of Reiki in his life.

thank

Christofer

CHRISTOPHER

One very cold January morning, I was called by Christopher's parents to his bedside in a hospital. He was suffering from a very rare form of leukaemia. He was dying.

His parents were waiting for me with anxiety, as a desperate attempt to save their beloved child's life. I told them not to hope about anything because I was not able to perform anything supernatural to save Christopher.

I knew that Christopher was going to leave his body. I knew I was going to do the best I could to put his soul at peace.

From the moment I entered the room, I saw a young man of about twenty five, who was looking at me in a very peaceful way. I will never forget the deepness of his eyes.

I could not perform a whole Reiki treatment on him, because I was not allowed to touch him.

I performed a distant Reiki treatment; I sat at the side of his bed without touching him, sending him loving angelic energy. I knew that Christopher was receiving it because his deep eyes, those of a very old soul ready to cross the bridge, became even more intense.

I treated him for a while. All of a sudden, Christopher started talking to me. Before then, there had been only eye contact. He said, "I know I am going to die, please bless my soul."

This was at the beginning of my mission as a Reiki Master and I was really overwhelmed by his request. I actually did not know what to say. Big tears starting coming out of my eyes and instinctively, I laid my hands on his head. He felt at peace and restful and I was filled with an interior peace that stayed with me for many months.

At the end of the Reiki, Christopher had a big smile on his face and I did too. I greeted him and left. I still have his words in my mind. As I was leaving the room, he repeated, "Thank you, Thank you."

I knew that I had to be there to help him crossing the bridge, after that experience I was called to many more deathbeds to give peace and rest to the dying. It is an honor that I cherish more than anything else.

Christopher left his body that night.

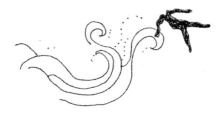

MARIA

MARIA

When Maria came to me, she had been wearing black for 10 years. This stunning Turkish woman had lost her son to throat cancer some years before our meeting. Since then, she had become a dead flower, the smile had gone from her face and she had withdrawn from life among the living. She did not want to live anymore.

When we first met I was really taken by her. I invited her to come and receive a Reiki treatment. I left it up to her. She was very stubborn. I remember her saying to me, "Why do you want to help me? Leave me alone. I do not deserve anything. I just want to die."

However, she soon found out that I was even more stubborn than she was. Gently, I continued to try to persuade her to come to one of our regular weekly meetings where she could receive Reiki not only from me but also from other students. Besides grieving for her lost son, Maria also suffered from Chronic Fatigue Syndrome, so she rarely left her home because she did not have the energy.

I finally persuaded her to have a treatment. I knew she would benefit a lot. During her first treatment, I could sense that some energy was moving; she got very emotional and after the treatment, we both cried for at least half an hour. I assured her that she would be okay, knowing in my heart that it would be a long but rewarding journey for both of us, working together.

I did not hear from Maria for a week, but when she finally called, she told me that she could not believe what she had experienced. All of a sudden, she had felt a boost of energy and she had been very active for days. Through the power of Reiki, Maria's subconscious mind began processing the grief she had held onto for so many years. Maria returned for more treatments, and as we continued to work together she started feeling better and had more energy. The once dead flower had come back to life again.

In the beginning, Maria always wore black. Gradually I convinced her to introduce new colors into her wardrobe. Colors are very important in our lives. I always talk about the importance of having colors around us, from what we eat, to what we wear and live in.

On my 35th birthday, I decided to have a farewell party because I was going to live in Colorado. I had invited all of my students. Maria was invited also. She was late, and I thought to myself, "She is very shy, I hope she comes."

When she arrived and entered the party, everybody turned to look at her. She was radiant in a very elegant dress of aqua, my favorite color. I was very proud. She had come out of her black tunnel of depression and Chronic Fatigue Syndrome. She was celebrating life now and wanted to help others. What a transformation! Seeing Maria in her lovely aqua dress, happy at last, was the most unforgettable present of all.

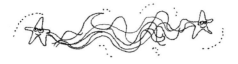

L VCA

LUCA

Luca is an interesting and joyful man. He is a top executive in a public firm. He works in human resources, and has a degree in biology. He is an acquaintance of mine.

He has never been interested in alternative therapies although he has been very attracted to everything that was strange and supernatural since he was a kid.

One day he was tormented by a back pain. He was tired and could not move. He called me up and asked me to do something about it.

I sent him distant Reiki. We decided that as his first treatment this would be very short, because Luca is a very vivacious man and he is not prone to sit or lay down relaxing for more than ten minutes. The treatment lasted just that time.

After ten minutes, his back pain had disappeared completely. He was extremely happy with the results. He was bending over and doing all kinds of movements that you cannot do if you have back pain. Everything had gone.

He realized that Reiki had helped him to feel more relaxed, melting those terrible knots in his back.

Often, he reminds me of that strange circumstance, as he calls it. He is now convinced that sometimes orthodox medicine can work together with the alternatives.

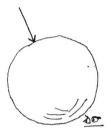

DIANA

Some years ago, in a health publication in England, appeared an article about Reiki, and how the Japanese healing had helped a woman come to terms with her abuse as a child and the things she had gone through since her childhood. After the publication of this article I was inundated by phone calls from men and women wanting to experience the same energy as the woman in the article.

There was a particular woman who got my attention.

Diana was a very nice English blonde woman. She was very successful in her business and wanted to make her long-term relationship with her husband work. She had been abused as a child and her fears of a man touching her had been with her for most of her life. She was now in her fifties and she still would not enjoy a good relationship with her husband because of those doubts.

I started working on her, explaining how important is for the chakras to spin in the right directions all the time.

I also explained to her that most people have fears in their mind and that Reiki works on the subconscious first, and when you are more relaxed inside yourself, the healing of the body comes naturally.

She seemed to understand my point.

I explained to her what I was going to perform, where my hands would be, and how relaxed she would feel.

I felt like Diana was absorbing all the energy she could. She was relaxing and her mind was calm and serene. This took a while before it all happened. I vividly remember her mind talking to me; when some people's eyes flicker all the time during a treatment, it is a sign that their minds are talking and finding it hard to relax. This was happening with Diana. She would come for a treatment and embrace the energy. Her healing process did not take long, she was feeling more in control, and more relaxed with her sexuality, she once told me that she had never felt like that before. Reiki was really helping the healing of old issues that she needed to address in her life.

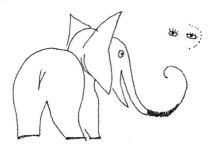

elaine

ELAINE

Reiki not only works on people but also on animals and plants.

Elaine is a beautiful Californian lady, of a beauty that it is at the same time elegant and wild. In her style she reminded me of a young Katharine Hepburn.

One day she called my office in Boulder, Colorado, where I was living in that period. She told me that one of my brochures had fallen on her feet and she did not know how and from where. She was looking for a Reiki Master and she realized that it was a signal.

Elaine booked a Reiki session. When she woke up after the treatment, she told me that was exactly what she was looking for in her life at that particular time.
I taught Reiki to her privately. Elaine was a loner and she did not want to take the course with a group.

At the end of the first level, she told me that she had the desire to practice Reiki on animals.

She told me that she had lived on a semi-deserted island with only animals and a small group of people until the island was evacuated and they had to leave. She was sad to leave the animals behind.

A few weeks later, Elaine was offered the opportunity to go to India. It was a gift from her mother.

When she got back, she came to tell me of her experiences and everything she had seen.

She was telling me that in India people use elephants to go from one side of town to the other. At night the pachyderms crashed on the ground from exhaustion. Elaine told me that she went to the animals, first from a distance and then closer, giving them soothing loving energy. She felt like the animals appreciated her love and compassion.

She told me that this had been a delightful experience for her heart.

She had learned that the dance that elephants do on Earth is the same that whales do in the sea. These beautiful dances allow Earth to be more balanced, and we need that a lot.

It is important that we treat animals with good manners, sending them unconditional love always. The strength of prayers and sending positive thoughts are the best things we can do to alleviate the suffering of people and animals all over the world.

If you go to a zoo, send animals loving thoughts. If you go to a circus, do the same. After all, those animals are only there for our enjoyment, I am sure they would rather be free in the jungle.
Elaine came back from India wanting to take Reiki II and learn how to send distant Reiki.

She is, today, one of my Reiki Master Teachers in US.

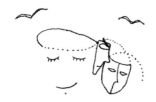

Thomas

THOMAS

Thomas, an actor, came to London for very delicate brain surgery. He was very distressed. One of my students asked me to go and see Thomas in the hospital. He had traveled from his native country to undergo this surgery.

I went to the hospital. I found Thomas to be an unpretentious person, although he was considered a God in his native country. He smiled at me with a most compassionate smile. I remember that I smiled back and I tried to comfort him for the operation he was going to have shortly. He was very tired and not speaking too much English. I visited Thomas several times prior to his surgery, performing Reiki primarily for comfort and to reassure him. Therefore, he would be mentally and spiritually prepared for the delicate procedure. After each treatment, he felt secure and loved and fell asleep.

During and after surgery, everything went well. My student and I continued to give him a Reiki treatment every day until he returned to his country. He recovered in half of the time the doctors had projected.

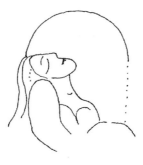

TULA

TULA

Tula was a beautiful Finnish woman who had been suffering from back pain for many years. She had given up her top executive job to undergo all sorts of treatments. Nothing seemed to help. She had always been attracted to metaphysical subjects.

One day she entered my center in London. She was in great pain. Years later, she told me she was guided to come and seek help. She knew that she had found a solution to her problems that day.

I began working on her. Usually if I have clients who suffer badly from pain, I see them for four consecutive times. The pain that had been in her back was spreading to her arms as well. The energy that was coming through for Tula was strong and powerful. She would usually fall asleep during the sessions. Soon, she started feeling relaxed and full of energy. Her pain began to vanish. Her life force returned and she began to feel happier. I could see her vibrant black eyes coming back to life. Reiki helped her mind to heal. Tula wanted to live, and through Reiki, her mind became stronger.

Tula asked me to train her in the practice of Reiki. Knowing that one day she would become a good and compassionate teacher, I agreed.

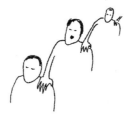

ANDRea

ANDREW

When I met Andrew, he was a man of about thirty-five years of age. He is a biologist and a naturalist, with the hobbies of traveling and photography.

He was an extremely skeptical and rational person. He did not believe in any of the alternative therapies.

One day he asked me for a Reiki treatment, because he liked the word Reiki. He enjoyed it so much that he decided to try a series of four. Each time, I would take him through a meditation to clear and balancing his chakras.

Andrew, slowly started to come to a deeper understanding of his capability to love himself, and every body else, unconditionally. He had a very strong and rational education, but slowly he was coming to terms with certain weaknesses inside himself. He could not accept anything that did not have a proper explanation that you couldn't scientifically prove.

In one of the sessions, for instance, he told me that an aunt of his used a gentle hand touch on his body whenever his was sick or did not feel well. His aunt was giving him Love. He felt well and energized each time.

Andrew today is one of my most brilliant students and he is approaching his third level of Reiki with enthusiasm and life joy.

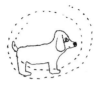

MANU

MANU (my dog)

In my book, I have told you that giving Reiki to people is the best gift of all, and I have also told you that pets and plants also benefit very well from Reiki. A cat or a dog will let you know when they are ready to receive a treatment.

Manu is a beautiful Golden Retriever from England. She is nine years of age but she still looks and acts like a puppy. Here is her beautiful story.

I knew that there was a special bond between me and this puppy since the moment I went to buy her from a kennel outside London. I had made arrangements with the owner of the litter for a female, and he told me: "Well, Mr. Vivo, I have only two females, so you had better hurry." I did. When I arrived there were five beautiful

Retrievers still being nurtured by their mother, and this one odd little puppy came toward me, clumsy and very sweet. I took her.

Manu proved to be a gentle and kind soul from the beginning. She was caring and kind. She would follow me everywhere I went, and she was growing up with the personality that would accompany her for the rest of her life.

When Manu was three years old I decided that I wanted her to have puppies. I took her to have eye and hip tests. She passed the eye test but unfortunately, she did not pass the hip test. The vet I was using at the time told me that Manu had a dysfunction in her hips and that she could not sustain a pregnancy because she would die during it. The vet also said that two of the bones in her hips were causing a middle bone to disintegrate, and that I would have to put her to sleep in a few months because she would begin limping and I would not want her to suffer.

I was distraught. I did not want to lose my adorable dog, and I certainly did not want to see her suffer. At that time, I had only my first degree Reiki. I started giving Reiki treatments to Manu daily. She loved it. She knew I was helping her with her suffering. She would lie down and, with a special sound, she would tell me, "Here I am, ready for you to give me Reiki." Therefore, I continued this for several months. Manu is now 9 years old; she has never limped, and she is a very happy and healthy dog.

She has a gentle, peaceful aura, which I know is the nature of Golden Retrievers anyway, but I am certain she is different now than before her Reiki treatment began. When I walk her, people ask me, "How old is your puppy?" I tell them she is no longer a puppy; she is nine years old and they can't believe it.

Her spirit and soul have been a gift from heaven to me. She is my teacher and my closest friend. If I am upset, she is the first one who comes to take care of me. It will always be this way for us.

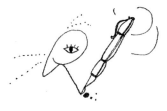

JANNE

JANNE

As a Reiki Master and a writer myself, my interaction with Janne affected me profoundly. She was an elderly French woman with a cancer that was destroying her fragile body. She had seen an ad about the healing effects of Reiki and decided to find a practitioner near her. We lived in the same neighborhood in London at that time. One day she stopped me in the supermarket to ask about Reiki. I was astonished that such an elderly woman would even know about Reiki, and at the same time I was happy because this was an indication that my dream for a global knowledge of Reiki seemed to be coming closer.

I invited Janne to my office that afternoon to offer her a treatment. I knew that something was wrong with her because she was so frail and obviously in a great deal of pain. I had seen her walking and pushing her shopping basket with very little inner force through my neighborhood, Chiswick, in London. She told me she was writing her memoirs of France during World War II, but her cancer was interfering with this important task.

As we became confidants, she started to tell me about her life in France and about the memoirs that she was writing. I clearly remember that one day she grabbed my arm and said, "I know you can help me. That is why I have come to you. You see, Mr. Vivo, I had to stop writing my memoirs because the cancer is eating my arm and I am not able to write anymore. But when I come to you for a treatment, and I go home, I can write another page of my book."

To the reader of my book I say this is the best reward that Reiki can give you. When you hear comments like this one, it opens your heart in a most wonderful and dramatic way. Reiki has the power to heal not only the person receiving treatments but also the Reiki practitioner giving the treatment. In this way, we further the healing of the entire planet. I will always be open to helping people through the universal love and beauty of Reiki.

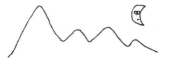

Kelly

KELLY

At the beginning of the ninety's I used to live in Paris, where I worked as a translator for an American computer firm. It was a pretty nice experience since I worked with people coming from all over the world. I became friends with Kelly, an intelligent American girl from NY. We used to talk a lot, to get to know one another, and our friendship grew closer and intimate.

The French experience finished. Kelly went back to US and I returned to London.

Kelly and I used to talk at least once a month, telling each other about our experiences and life. Kelly had moved to San Diego, California, where her brother lived.

A few years went by and I was deciding to leave London for a while to go and live in the US. I did not know where to go or which state to choose from. The reply to my question came suddenly one morning.
Kelly called me from Colorado, with terrible news; doctors had

told that she had cancer of the ovaries. My decision was made; I would go to where Kelly lived to give her all my support and love.

So I did.

I was very pleased to begin a new life where I did not know anyone but Kelly.
As a Reiki Teacher, I am always in search of new experiences that can expand my knowledge and my spiritual path. I have changed my place of residence so many times that I could have spread my Reiki teachings in many corners of the planet.

Arriving in Colorado and meeting Kelly again after so many years gave me a sense of great joy and understanding. At the same time, a stab to my heart at confronting the girl I had met in Paris years before, so full of life and joy; now replaced with the woman in front of me, defenceless and thin, with long grey hair.

Kelly and I spoke a lot; we were famous for being on the phone for hours, even from one continent to the other. Once I moved closer, we used to meet and have long and relaxing walks on the Rocky Mountains.

Once we took some stale bread and some nuts, and Kelly took me to a forest where there was a colony of prairie dogs that she used to feed daily. It was amazing seeing these wild animals gathering around Kelly when she arrived with food.

During our walks, Kelly used to tell me about her life; her difficult relationship with her father, whom she did not get along with, and had been verbally abusive for years. She had a big fear of being with men.

In Reiki we believe that if our mind gives us signals of fear, or fragility, sooner or later our body will experience some kind of turmoil.

Kelly was afraid of being with a man and she developed a cancer of the ovaries that had expanded all over her body.

I used to give her Reiki often to soothe her pains. Sometimes her ache was so strong that she did not like to be touched.

Kelly died in a cold January evening, leaving me with much grief and sadness. She left me with the awareness that we should listen to ourselves and our voice within at all times.

Kelly also made me promise to reveal her story to the world, so I did.

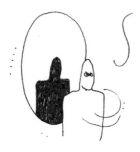

GISELVA

GISELA

Gisela was a Hungarian woman I met once I moved to Boulder Colorado.

She was a stunningly beautiful woman who had been under a lot of stress. She had decided that she wanted to home school her two children. She did not have a job and I knew that she was struggling financially.

She came to me after seeing my picture in a local paper.

She had heard about Reiki and made an appointment for a treatment. Later she told me she wanted to learn the ancient Japanese healing technique.
Gisela told me that she was a tachycardia sufferer and that she might not be ready for the treatment. I told her to relax, empty her mind

for a while, and forget her worries.

She lay on the treatment table and sure enough, as soon as I put my hands on her head her heartbeat started going very fast. She could not take it, she had to get up so I continued to give her Reiki while she was seated on the table.

She felt more relaxed and peaceful after the treatment, so she continued to come for more sessions.

The second time she came, she was feeling very nervous. As soon as I started working on her though, she relaxed and went to sleep. She confessed to me later that she had not felt so relaxed in many years. She was now comfortably lying on the table for the whole duration of the treatment.

Gisela knew that I was teaching a Reiki I class and she asked me whether I thought she was ready to learn. I never discourage people who want to learn Reiki; I know that Reiki is a very helpful modality for the soul. I told her that she could take my class.

She took Reiki I. The harmony in the class was exquisite.

Gisela was happy. She agreed that her tachycardia was better and that she could now give Reiki to herself and to her children daily.

One day, Gisela called me in Italy, where I was teaching some courses, to tell me that she had to have a hernia operation. She told me that she was not scared at all and that she would use Reiki during surgery.

A few days later, I called from Italy to ask her husband how she was doing, and by surprise, she was already at home, schooling her children. I was surprised. She told me that she did not stay in the hospital and she never had the anesthesia, she had given herself Reiki all the time during the surgery and that she felt very relaxed and very at peace. The doctors had performed an operation on her while she was awake. She said that she was thinking of me all the time, visualizing my face in front of her, and that had relaxed her more and more. I was mesmerized and apparently, the doctors were too.

Gisela and her family are among a group of people who continued to support, help, and encourage my work and my studies of Reiki while I was living in Boulder.

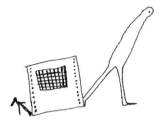

GIovANNI

GIOVANNI

I was in my home in London one evening, some years ago. I was in my therapy room, writing notes on the people I had seen that day, and the ones I would be seeing the following one. It was raining cats and dogs, and I was sipping hot tea, I had opened the doors of the veranda to smell the wet grass. I could see a beautiful fox, not rare in the English gardens, looking around the yard.

It was a magnificent evening. I was playing some relaxing music in the background. I was calm; enjoying the evening and thinking of a particular client I had seen that afternoon.

Giovanni was an Italian Reiki student of mine who had come from a small village in Sicily to London to look for a job. He had been my last patient that afternoon, and I felt like he wanted to talk more. I was right. Giovanni told me that he wanted to tell me the story of his life. I asked him if he was sure, and he said that yes he wanted to tell me, because he was sure that I would understand him with no judgement. So it was.

Since his mother had died, Giovanni felt very lonely; he had left one brother, one sister, and his father back home, but he had never had a good relationship with his dad.

His father was a very strict man, with his own ideas and closed in his own world. These ideas clashed with Giovanni's. His mother, on the other hand, had been his friend and his confidante all along. Intuitively, Giovanni knew how bad his parent's relationship was; how many things his mother had to swallow all her life. Once his mother died the solid family structure died too.

Giovanni had come to see me and together we had done Reiki therapy on forgiveness and healing. That is why then he decided to open up to me; forgiving his father, his mother, and himself.

There are a lot of people who hold grudges for things happened in the past or against people who are not here anymore. We cannot go forward in life while creating more regrets and revenge; we do not solve anything doing so. We only need to project love, to give love, to send love; forgiving ourselves first, and others around us. If we are able to forgive, we will create a peaceful world around us and we will be in harmony with everybody and everything.

In the world where we are living, one of the most important things is forgiveness. I know it is very difficult, but it is vital nowadays, and we can do it, with patience and joy from the heart. In doing so, life will smile back on us.

Giovanni had told me that since childhood, he felt like the odd one. He did not understand the world around him. He felt that everyone around him was like Martians from other planets.

He would tell me about his intuitions and his perceptions, and how he had created an unreal world, where everything was allowed, with love and light.

Giovanni was an introverted timid, closed child, and people thought he had serious psychological problems. He did not like the things and games that appealed to the children of his age. He liked to look at the world with different eyes; to look at nature, defenceless animals, and people who need help and hope.

One day, Giovanni's father, one of those macho Southern Italian men, decided that things had to change. Giovanni needed to become a real man. He took his child to see a psychiatrist. The therapy took twelve long years. It did not help Giovanni at all. His doctor was a very religious one and each time Giovanni would tell him about ideas, perceptions, intuitions, he would tell him to go to church and confess his sins.

Giovanni was not a very good pupil at school either. He was suffering so much inside and he was bullied at school and had a very strict and nasty teacher who would beat him up almost every day. He considered school to be like a prison. He felt lonely and miserable, finding protection only at home with his mother and his sister, with whom he could talk and live comfortably. His father was never at home; he was working all the time and never had time for his kids.

For all these reasons Giovanni decided to create his secret world; dreaming with his eyes open about going away forever, flying like his angels had told him.

At the age of thirty five Giovanni came to see me with a big desire to change. He had started attending my Reiki Exchanges and then decided to come for Reiki Treatments in my office.

The Reiki Exchanges are monthly meetings I have with my students, to give Reiki to people who needed it, and for the practice of the students themselves.

As I have said many times before, I do not believe in long therapies; we do not need more than eight treatments to energetically clear someone's body. Giovanni was shocked, thinking that he had been in therapy for so many years without solving anything. I tried to explain to him that since he had come to receive Reiki at this particular moment in his life, it meant that unconsciously he was committed to heal and forgive.

We began the therapies. The first ones were quite painful, and then bit by bit his fears started to vanish, like his inadequacy towards his family and relatives. He began to tell me that he did not feel so insecure anymore. He had started talking to his father again, looking straight in his eyes. He also told me that from time to time that fear came back to him. Each time that happened he would put his hands on the heart chakra to center himself, and that would immediately give him a sense of peace and relaxation.

Giovanni told me with sadness that he had always looked for his father approval. It never happened.

His father used to praise Giovanni's siblings all the time. Giovanni had never been hugged by his father and never in his life had he been told nice words of encouragement, not even for the difficult and brave choices he had made in his life.

I advised Giovanni to forgive his father and go forward. Maybe Giovanni's father was very proud of him but just did not know how to show it. Giovanni was the one who had left home and not followed his father's business as the other two had done.

Giovanni decided to study Reiki because he felt like he could improve his life.

Reiki is Love

I know that today he is a great Reiki Master Teacher.

He spreads the Universal Energy in many corners of the planet.

I will never stop saying that Reiki is Only Universal Love. Millions of people practicing Reiki are energetic channels who give universal love to everyone who needs it; in doing so, we find ourselves in a better world, with peace, brotherhood, and respect for animals and nature.

Earth vibrations are speeding very fast. I say, forgive and forget. Open your heart and fly. Do not look back, look forward, to the enchanting future that we all have before us.

Gaetano Vivo

"THE SOUL CANNOT LIVE WITHOUT A POEM"

ARISTOTELES

"*I called a swallow: solidarity and I asked it to fly,*
There, in that place, where there is no peace,
I sent my swallow to bring the light.
It helped the children feeding the poorest;
It helped the women.
There, in that place, where there is no peace
It restored a smile."

FLAVIA

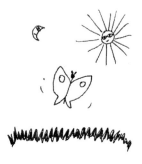

BRUNA

BRUNA

Reiki has changed my life. It is only a distant thought; that feeling of anguish and impotence, when I struggled with my worries, feeling that I was the only one on Earth to have gigantic problems.

It is also only a thought; that terrible headache that lived with me for years, making my life miserable and sad.

Here I am now, writing my story and getting emotional at remembering all this; as they say; writing heals all emotions. I have now a different strength inside me that pushes me every day of my life. If I feel weak, sad, and alone I know that the energy of Reiki will be with me forever. Nowadays, I speak about energy. I let my coworkers know what I am doing, they see a different light in my eyes, a different way of approaching life, and they see a big change happening inside me.

Reiki is Love

I celebrate my love for the energy by starting the day with a self Reiki treatment, I am certain that this allows me to go forward through the many worries that I have during the day. Before, I would cry, I would despair, I would criticize; now, I smile, I fight, and I forgive.

Today I appreciate a sunset, a dawn, the sea, a child's smile. Reiki has taught me all these things. Reiki is Love.

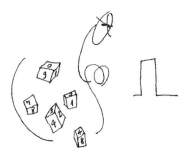

GERTRUDE

GERTRUDE

Reiki has changed my life forever. It has given me a great balance.

I am a teacher of mathematics in a scientific high school; my life runs between numbers, problems, and rationality. I have approached Reiki in a very difficult moment of my life, in which I was called upon to initiate some important and upsetting choices.

Thanks to Reiki, I left forever medicines and therapists and I have discovered my capacity and myself: I became more decisive and I have no fear of confronting changes.

I have succeeded to better manage relationships with others and to make my points of view known, without experiencing the worthlessness that has marked my life so far.
I continue to be available to others without canceling my whole

personality in the process. I understand that if I am well and peaceful inside, I can give love and happiness to others.

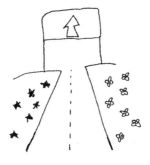

PILAR

PILAR

When I decided to take the first level, I was not aware that I would travel so far.

At the beginning, I was frightened and very insecure as to how I could use Reiki. I was not sure I could use it on others or myself, but at the same time I was very curious about the changes that were happening to me. After the first level, taken with a teacher in Spain where I reside, I waited for almost two years before taking the second level. I had already decided to continue this route but I did not find the right teacher for me. When I met Gaetano everything came so natural; getting to know him, to speak with him, to confide in him, it was as though I had known him forever.

Naturally, he has given me the force to find myself, to trust myself, and the courage to go forward in this spiritual journey.

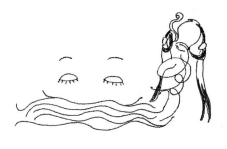

TIZIANA

TIZIANA

I have approached this natural healing method with lots of enthusiasm.

After the first attunement, I had a new energy to run inside myself. With my eyes shut, I could cherish each moment of the sacred ritual. I was able to fly in other dimensions, carried out from the teacher's musical voice and energy, feeling in peace with the entire universe and myself, experiencing unimaginable emotions, seeing colors and attractive landscapes. Calling upon the angels who look after me, I imagined that my deceased husband and parents were there with me. From time to time, I felt like they were whispering in my ears words of optimism and encouragement to go forward in this path.

Everybody can learn Reiki. The teacher re-opens your channels. We are all born with our channels wide open, and then they close while we grow up. If you then decide to start a spiritual journey, you will have your channels re-open to get the universal life energy flowing through you.

Undoubtedly, in these last years my life has improved a lot, now I am in a better mood all the time and with a great sense of peace inside myself.

Treating myself every morning, I enter into contact with the real me, myself, learning to listen to myself, to love me more.

In this world where self-centeredness and selfishness prevail, I like to stop, reflect, and ponder. I succeed in the most difficult things and face life with more delight.
This is the real gift that Reiki has given me.

I have now undertaken the path for the third level, I know that will be long and binding but surely will continue to make me grow to make me appreciate the beauty of life and to make me surpass the obstacles that inevitably I will meet, with force and serenity.

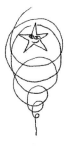

SONYA

SONYA

Meeting Reiki has meant, for me, to radically upset my person and my entire universe. When I understood that, I found that was what I actually was looking for; to change my person, to balance my spiritual being, to grow as a woman.

The chaos was total; all of the negative aspects of my personality were leaving me forever. All those aspects that Sonya had been working on for years; hiding behind some calm and tolerant way of living that nonetheless had been better to fight there and then.
It was almost a year ago that I put Reiki into practice. I have learned to help others, to alleviate their deep down pains. Learning Reiki has made me understand that I am a human being and as such, I have limitations beyond which it is not always possible to go, but to learn to accept them, to coexist with them, to love them.
This is who I am today, always the same, but with a large certainty: I cannot know what the future holds. I can only live in the present.

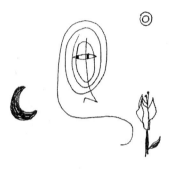

FIORELLA

FIORELLA

Reiki has shown me the road that I have always consciously and unconsciously sought. Before my pathology took me to live the experience of the coma, I had always asked myself the reason why and what was the message to learn from it.

After the experience that life has given me, I have begun to see events of daily life in a different way. It seems like my sensibility is growing and with it an emotional feeling towards other people.

These changes occurred in my life from the first approach I had with Reiki. It has been a lot simpler to reach a greater balance and self-knowledge, and to understand how I can be of use to others. Communicating, to infuse calm, and give love, in every day of my life.

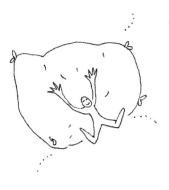

BARBARA

BARBARA

My spiritual journey has begun attending the first level of Reiki in October 2002. Subsequently I received the second level.

I have always been a special child, so people say. I think that my gifts have started broadening ever since my father tried to kill my mother with rat's poison; she drank it, and she was in a bad shape for quite sometime. She is good now, and we study Reiki together. They say that if you have something that happens to you in an early age, this will allow you to grow faster and with special gifts, this is not always the case, but it is in my case. The benefits of Reiki on me and my family have been great and I have verified them during school exams, tests, and dealing with my life's issues.

I am only twenty three.

I hear my guardian angels. I talk to them. I know that they are always with me when I go to bed at night, protecting me during my sleep.

I helped my grandmother who was constantly in bed with her pains. She is now with the angels, and I also feel her around me.

I clear the house from negative energies. Reiki is helping me to understand the crazy world in which we are living, to broaden and to go beyond, to understand people and try to give them love.

I have much belief in God and above all in Jesus Christ. They granted me the privilege of receiving the gift of Reiki, and I think they have created good situations for me to meet my teacher. I am still very young but I thank, and I will always thank, the celestial forces that allowed me to arrive at this point and beyond.

This is my story, written for all those people that see Reiki with suspicion or with a lot of scepticism and to those people I say: "Open your heart and your mind, cultivate your spirit, and above all love everyone!"

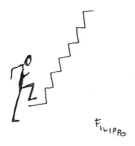

Filippo

FILIPPO

It has been since my adolescence that I was considered the different one. I had been drawn towards the peculiar, the alternative; an interest that I have not cultivated because I was too distracted by the materialism of daily life.

At the age of twenty-seven, I started hearing the word Reiki almost everyday. Then it was pronounced from my favourite singer on national television. She was speaking on how Reiki had changed her life.
I immediately started researching material on Reiki and who was offering seminars in my area.

I absolutely knew that this had to be my spiritual path. I was desperately looking for a teacher. The choice was vast and not always I felt like Reiki was only love. There was a lot of speculation, a lot of people being in competition on who was offering the best seminar and why.

One day I was invited to go to a free lecture hosted by Gaetano Vivo, it was love at first sight. My wife and I felt beautiful energies coming from this man, from the experiences he was talking about in his life with Reiki. We decided to sign up for his workshop then and there.

The seminar, which lasted a weekend, was of a deeper healing happening all over my body and mind. A bad back pain that had lived with me for the past ten years had been transformed into joy to begin a new day with enthusiasm and energy.

I had received the gift to look inside myself and the knowledge of the infinite possibilities given to me from a higher source. Since then I have begun to give Reiki to all the people around me, friends and relatives who, initially sceptical, have tried the benefits of Reiki, changing radically their ideas and their convictions.

The greatest gift is to send absent Reiki to people all over the globe, staying comfortably seated in your living room. Reiki makes you feel useful, spreading our loving energy wings to the ones who are suffering and are far from us all.

The three week purification we go through after the first Reiki level is very strong and debilitating, the energy in your body keeps changing until you are balanced, physically and mentally.

To my knowledge, I can certainly say that Reiki has been the chosen path; someone higher than myself has chosen this incredible healing technique for me to be healed forever and to help others through me.

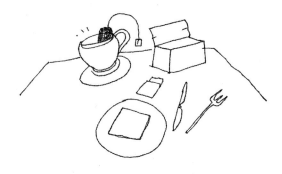

RAFFAELLA

RAFFAELLA

My childhood was not a happy one, because of some diseases that have beaten my body since birth.

At eighteen, a terrible asthma debilitated me completely.

Then a nice period, I met my husband and got married, had a child, and for the first time understood what happiness was. It did not last long...at twenty-three, I knew the deep pain and tearing at the loss of my mother: a breast cancer took her away forever. I suffered and prayed, but also cursed against an impotent God that appeared to me so cruel and that gave my family only pain and grief.
After ten years my father died. I had thought that with my mother's death nothing could have hurt me more, I was wrong. I felt like God had taken away my roots, my deepest part. After a few years I was diagnosed with cancer myself; I felt like I knew it all along.

I started some very painful therapies, and most importantly an interior journey. I knew that deep down a change was occurring. I started approaching alternative therapies, reading books on such subjects that could expand my knowledge. A word got my full attention: Reiki.

I felt an attraction towards this word but I did not know where to find someone who would teach me. Then, on a health publication, I read an article about Reiki and Gaetano Vivo, and my life changed. I took Reiki I & II. The technique let all my "ghosts" emerge from my past, Mr. Vivo took my hand and, as he does with everybody, showed me the way of deep awareness. Reiki has transformed me and continues to do so. Some health issues persist, but I now have a key on how to approach them. Moreover, I have reached a psychological and mental balance that gives me inner serenity.

One of the most beautiful results that I have achieved with Reiki so far is with one of my pupils, who suffered from depression caused from the unexpected death of his uncle. His parents, after several attempts to help him, surrendered since the boy had fallen in a state of total panic. I spoke to them about Reiki and I offered him a treatment. They accepted at once, even though they had to overcome the hostility of some relatives who, being doctors, absolutely did not believe in these types of treatments, much less in the Reiki, which they did not know anything about.

After the first treatment, Flaviano said that he was feeling more relaxed and calm, and with the passing of the days, it was him who asked me for a Reiki treatment. After a month, the boy was completely recovered.

Reiki is Love

He had regained his strength, was going out with his friends, studying, and enjoying his young life.

This experience made me understand that there are events still not comprehensible to our rational mind, which we must accept with great humility; moreover, it has reached the truer, deeper, and authentic part of me, giving me an increasing ability to communicate with others and allowing my conscience to expand. Reiki has healed the wounds of my mind and I have learned to love again, everybody, and to all I give a smile and my heart.

I will never stop thanking Gaetano Vivo for everything he has done for me and the horizons that he has opened wide before my eyes. I want to dedicate to him this poem by Pablo Neruda:

> *Protect the shadow in order to see it from dusk*
> *We reach out and touch the walls,*
> *We spy the light in order to catch it*
> *And once and for all the sun of every day belongs to us.*

Thanks, Gaetano, thanks from the depth of my heart. Thanks to you, I can watch the sun again.

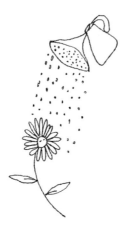

CATHERINE

CATHERINE

I have great respect for Reiki. After the first time my Reiki Master back home gave me a treatment, I knew that I had really felt the most pure form of love. I not only felt a deep mental change, but also a physical one. I had never before felt like my mind and body were working so closely together. After I left her house that first time I felt like I had been reborn. I had a tendency, for days, to touch my lips, as if I was feeling them for the first time. I was able to look deeply into a person's eyes as he talked to me, without making them or myself at all uncomfortable. I could feel energy radiating from my hands, head, and abdomen, at the same time I felt completely grounded. Breathing was easy and felt beautiful. I could feel the energies in my body realigning. After the Reiki treatment, I could not eat anything unhealthy or be around cigarettes or alcohol without becoming uncomfortable. My body felt pure and it needed purity. As someone gives me a Reiki treatment or I give myself or someone else Reiki, I have intense feelings of love, kindness, patience, understanding, and calm.

This is what I felt when I left Mr Vivo's office. It is now three days later and I still feel such a profound difference from the way I felt before coming to see you. It is really quite amazing. Many times, I have been told in my life that I am calming to be around. After being around me for a short while I often have people say thing like "It is so easy to be around you, I haven't felt this relaxed in a while." After receiving a Reiki treatment I always notice that this tendency increases. Leaving my Reiki friend at home was difficult, because I wanted to learn all that I could from her about Reiki and healing. However, moving to Colorado and coming to school was the right thing to do, I can feel it. I waited for about two months and then decided I wanted to find someone in Colorado to guide me in studying Reiki. This is when I called you. I am glad to have met you and I am looking forward to getting to know you.

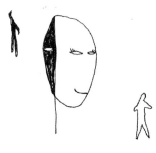

Elle

ELLE

In order to explain how and why Reiki has worked its magic and transformed my life I need to explain a little about my personal "history"........I was born with dislocated hips and had four major operations at three years old. My parents divorced when I was eight, due to my father having an affair with my mum's best friend. Their divorce was extremely bitter and obviously deeply hurtful for my brother and I. My mother got custody of us so we lived with her and as the failed marriage had torn her to shreds, she ceased to be a mother and behaved like a young, "free," single woman, constantly telling us kids we were "wicked" and disloyal, very much leaving us alone in the evenings to fend for ourselves.

I had a passion for the theatre and lived out my dreams by singing my head off in the lounge when no-one was around. At fourteen, I was cast in a major role in a big West End show, but just as contracts were exchanged they found out how young I was and had to withdraw the contract as it would have been illegal for me to continue. Showbiz, hey?! Things back at home with my mum grew steadily worse and I always felt forced to swap roles with her and ensure that her volatile mood swings didn't get too out of control. However, one night when I was fifteen she threw a major tantrum and I pinned her down by her shoulders on the bed while she kicked and bit and screamed that I didn't know how lucky I was. She told me that when she was my age she had been raped by her step-father. Now what can one say to that? So I very calmly let go of her, stood up and walked out. That night I moved in with my father and my step-mother and couldn't actually see my mum for the next two years. I moved to the capital with no money, no support, and no address to go to. I started drama school and also started going out with boys.

Needless to say my relationships were not exactly healthy and over the course of the next ten years although my acting career took off, my personal life was a disaster, involving two abortions along the way. What I'm trying to explain is; I had a lot to heal!

Then along came an angel who knew I was short of money and offered to teach me Reiki, completely free of charge. During the lunch hour of my Reiki I course I wrote in my diary, "This day will change my life." Little did I know then just how true an insight I had been given. Through the gentle guidance of my wonderful Reiki Master I discovered that actually I was not this "wicked" person I had always assumed I was.

I discovered that although my mother hadn't physically abused me or my brother, she had certainly abused us emotionally. Every time we achieved something she undermined us by "raping" our confidence and the shame we felt from her being involved with much younger men is indescribable. At the time I felt very close to my father who was totally unemotional and any time I was upset he would point at the T.V and say, "What have you got to be upset about? Look at those poor kids in Ethiopia. They've got real problems." I did feel terribly sorry for those children but everything is relative and their situation did not negate my world falling apart when my parents split. At this point I should say that both my mum and dad had obviously gone through a difficult time and they weren't *all* bad. I am extremely grateful for their better qualities, which have certainly given me and my brother strength in life. However, as I said before, I needed a lot of healing.....

I feel Reiki is unique because when you are attuned it's almost as if you admit to yourself and the Universe that you cannot continue living with so much pain in your heart, your mind, your spirit, or your body. Reiki brings such incredible healing at such a deep "soul level," its power is rooted in gentleness, for the self and others. When you physically touch someone you meet them at soul level and their "history" doesn't matter. One human to another you offer yourself as a channel for pure, unconditional love. Nothing is forced - the person decides whether they wish to release their pain or, if the time is not right, to hang on to it until they're ready. There is no ego involved. Only love. Also, one doesn't need to talk, although often things come up during a treatment or class. Old memories perhaps that need cleansing and clearing, freeing you to become the person you were always meant to be. REIKI has allowed me to make peace with myself, my folks, and my past and has encouraged me to take full responsibility for my life without playing the "victim."

I feel blessed to have met my extraordinary Reiki Master for he has shown me how to shine and become the beautiful flower I hid inside. I now practise and teach Reiki and unconditionally love myself and everybody else! Reiki really has transformed my life. Please let this true healing system bring you happiness, joy, and fulfilment. A new life beckons...

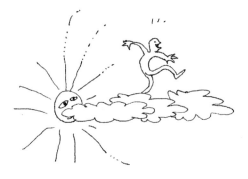

CARLA

CARLA

My name is Carla, I am forty-five and I am a schoolteacher. My first approach with Reiki was when I was offered a treatment for my back pain. I had suffered from it for many years.

After only one treatment, my back pain disappeared completely.

I was feeling like a butterfly. This has been the motivating force that has pushed me to learn Reiki. I knew that this particular technique would take me very far, and it has. The state of well-being that I had acquired during the treatment lasted for days after, and this is yet another of the fantastic things of the Reiki treatment.

What is Reiki? It is only Love, to give to everybody; Reiki is a smile, a caress, a touch, giving love to all beings.

I constantly give Reiki to my cats and my plants, and you can always feel a sense of calm and tranquility in the house. The energy of Reiki creates wonderful things.

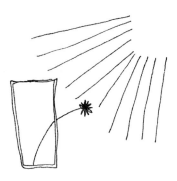

TOMMASO

Reiki is an extraordinary system that allows the healer to be connected to the universal energy, perceiving it like unconditional Divine Love, supporting all wonders of creation.
A Reiki treatment harmonizes the four bodies (physical, ethereal, astral, mental) acting on the chakras in order to balance them. Imposing your hands and transmitting universal energy and unconditional love gives the person a tool to look inside in a deeper way for healing.

My personal experience with Reiki, begun in June 2001 with a combined course of first and second level, in which I participated with great enthusiasm in order to give answers to some fundamental questions of my life. I learned the self-Reiki techniques and the one of treating others. I began to give Reiki to myself every day. With the passing of the days, I was not only healing my physical body from those small dysfunctions that I had (colitis, gastritis), but I was changing my way to observe and to perceive the world.

At the beginning, I found again a balance with nature: the tree's energy, the sea's sound, the smell of the salt from the sea, getting warmed by a sun beam, which I now see not only as a source of heating the planet but as a source of balancing the solar plexus of the planet and us.

My new optimism helped me with my relationship with my relatives, friends, and coworkers. Looking at other's inner beauty and discovering nice people around me. Currently I am deepening my acquaintance of Reiki with treatments on people and above all attending a course of third level. I am discovering every day that Reiki is a truly wonderful inner and evolutionary journey. It is helping me healing my fears, my traumas, my anxieties, and worries connected to my conscious and unconscious mental structures.

Today I have understood profoundly that if we want to help ourselves in a definite way, without incurring in the same mistakes, we must have the courage to watch ourselves deeply inside facing our shadow self and healing it in the process, carrying them to the light.

We must purify our being to be able to be a pure channel of Universal Energy, consecrating our life to the universal Love. In truth, we can irradiate this love to the entire humanity with the certainty that our presence, also silent, will be able to give others great blessings.

NINA

NINA

I like to talk about Reiki as my emotional rebirth. I realize that from that first lesson, my life started slowly changing forever.
Fortunately, I did not suffer from any serious problems, but I lived surrounded by people who oppressed me, took me for granted, and abused my friendship and my generosity.
I was like a sponge, absorbing everybody's problems which then left me completely deprived of my energy. The so called "energy vampires."
I now know how to protect myself, it is very simple, and I visualize universal energy surrounding me from head to toe.

People look at me in a different light nowadays, they say I give out a lot, but I am never tired or nervous about it. I know that Reiki protects me from bad vibrations and lower energies.

Reiki looks inside me with clarity and love. Learning Reiki has transformed my life.

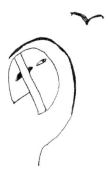

FLAVIO

FLAVIO

My path towards the expansion of Love.

I think the history of my inner change does not start from today, but a few years ago. In 1987, my life seemed to be flowing magnificently: a beautiful job, a pretty and affectionate wife, a wonderful child, a cozy little house, a new car, and many friends. All of a sudden, all this changed for the worst. I began having serious psychological problems, dissatisfaction, worries, I did not feel like going to work anymore, I only wanted to be shut in the house and see no one.
I refused to go out of the house or go to work if not accompanied. More than two years went by and my wife, tired of this, decided to get a divorce. I was in a limbo. I did not feel like going to the psychiatrist anymore and I completely shut myself inside.

One day, a friend told me about somebody who arranged trips to India to see a guru, this same person organized weekly meditation classes at her house. Out of curiosity I attended one of these evenings with my wife, who was also in a desperate situation for the premature loss of her mother. Both of us were mesmerized by the effect of that evening. We enjoyed going there every week, praying, and chanting. Soon I discovered that something was wrong with them, I felt manipulated and obsessed and left the circle. My wife, however, still enjoyed them, going to India once or twice a year.

Those meetings broadened my horizons; I started reading books on different spiritual subjects, going to lectures and exhibitions of Natural Healing Methods. In one of these, I met Gaetano Vivo.
I had been looking everywhere to learn Reiki, as I had read many books on the subject. At his booth, Gaetano invited us to a free lecture on Reiki a few days later. I went along and became interested in the universal love energy and its effects on people. Mr. Vivo gives his lectures having a group of his students always present to demonstrate what he talks about. We were asked to receive a little demonstration of Reiki, and the effects on me were incredible. I was in a deep state of well-being and peace, I felt like I had been taken by an angel. I had feelings that I cannot describe in words. I felt the presence of a guardian angel. Following that experience, I decided to take Reiki I & II, and that has been a growing acquaintance of this wonderful planet of Reiki.

Today, I am a Reiki Master; it seems like living a fantastic, indescribable adventure. My life is now completely different. This is my story; a story of changes, of an inner spiritual evolution.

I thank God every day for having met my Reiki master, a truly highly spiritual being on this planet today who teaches only Reiki from his beautiful Heart.

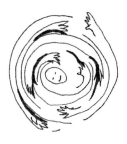

OMAR

OMAR

I am fifty; I am in a continuous spiritual search that gives serenity to my existence. I have been teaching Yoga for many years for the pleasure of doing it. In real life, I am a hairdresser. Reiki has crossed my road many times; I had never taken it into consideration to take a course.

I still remember the words of a famous guru: "If you are looking for water, avoid making many attempts, digging small wells here and there, focus on digging a deep one. You will have more possibilities of being successful." My fear was that Reiki was a small well and nothing else. The last years have been of no inspirations to me and teaching Yoga did not give me any more satisfaction; I was looking for new ideas.

One day, I met two people in the center where I teach yoga. They came to give a demonstration of Reiki treatments. Those two people did not know that thanks to them, my light started to brighten up and heat my soul again. When I saw them performing Reiki, I knew deep down that they had left a clear mark inside me. One of those two people became my Reiki Master.

Taking Reiki I, old pains and issues have come up. I have lived various experiences, like a late morn for my mother's death, or like a light touch as a caress that was pampering my body, like they were operating on me different sensations and touches.

I am convinced that when we give Reiki, we are not alone. We work together with spirit guides and angels who help us in the process.

I know now for sure that Reiki is not one of those small wells that the guru was talking about, but a great tool to heal our soul.

I thank God, for having helped me finding Reiki as an extra tool in my infinite search for spirituality.

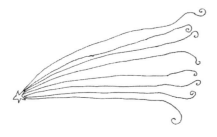

drubalkns

THE RAINBOW

RAINBOW is all around me.

Words are sometime so little to describe what I feel today.
Reiki has shown me the way to re-discover, indeed reawaken new feelings inside me, it made the more hidden perceptions emerge.
This journey started several years ago, when I was looking for something that could improve life.
I started seeing the light, like following a comet, and here I am again following it, a star of unconditional love and light towards me and others.
Thanks for having entered my life. Thanks from the depths of my heart.

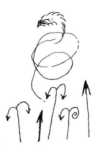

Stella

STELLA

After the complications of a chronic disease, the Systemic Lupus Erythematosus, I developed a "Lupic Pneumonia," which gave me a series of respiratory difficulties sending me in a deep coma for five days. It has been an unforgettable experience, because I am here today to talk about it, and for the feelings and emotions, that were given to me unconsciously. One of those feelings was the one of lightness and freedom from my body that was flying like a feather in the sky. It felt like my soul had reached the highest point of its evolution. These feeling will remain in my mind forever.

Other less pleasant sensations were seeing the suffering of other people in the same reanimation room to where I was, fighting for their lives; I saw some of them leaving and most of them coming back to earth. My experience ended in a somewhat traumatic way, because I lived the moment of the return with a disagreeable feeling and nostalgia, leaving the beauty of lightness and feeling heavy in my body again. The convalescence last three long months.

Many times, I think about what happened. The coma experience made me looking around in a better way, looking at the people who suffer differently.

After this experience, my life has completely changed and I feel I am now a better person. I no longer fear death, I do not see it like the end of everything, like a place of suffering, or a black hole; death is life, it is a passage in a new dimension, a new journey that is about to start.

Four more years passed, and while managing a bookstore, I happened to read a book on Reiki. My life was changing again.

Reiki, for me, is a new awareness. A new path that everyone should follow and should appreciate for its simplicity and for the love we can give to everyone.

This new path has given me the strength to go forward in life, giving me the opportunity of being closer to my beloved father while he was passing, knowing that he was going to a better place with no pain and no suffering.

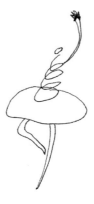

VI OVA

VIOLA

My experience with the Reiki began by reading your book, published in Italy, "Risveglia il tuo cuore col Reiki." Since then, I felt a strange feeling towards the subject, and an odd energy pervading my being.
I felt a strong drive inside to take the first level because I wanted to heal myself of a myoma. Doctors had advised me to have it surgically removed.

I remember that the weekend after the Reiki I level, I was scheduled to go to the hospital for an echography. Each time I had gone to have that test, the myoma had gotten larger and larger; that morning to my surprise, the myoma was few millimeters smaller. I thought, "It is the Reiki."

I can only say, that since the Reiki course I feel different inside, calmer and less anxious. I work for an airline and the level of stress is overwhelming all the time, especially in this time and age.
I now have a tool that allows me to relax and feel more comfortable within myself and when feel ready helping others.
After Reiki, I have met people whom I had not seen for years, and all of them have told me how much I have changed, and that I had a different light in my eyes.

I am so glad I have met Reiki, something that I had been looking for, for a long time.

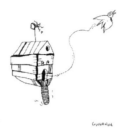

THE FAMOUS SINGER

My story began some years ago in the beautiful city of Milan. In that period I was living there, as I was a daily guest in a National television show. I was meeting important people for my career and my success as a singer. I had never participated in a television show, so this was my first experience and I was really enjoying it. I felt like I was in a fairytale. I had great projects for my future like the future Ella Fitzgerald.

One day, all of a sudden, I was diagnosed with a cancer to the thyroid; I had a little ball of five centimetres on my throat. The darkness surrounded me.

The doctors said that the ball had to be removed with surgery; there was nothing else we could have done. They needed to understand the nature of the tumour, whether it was benign or malignant. I continued to sink in more darkness; because the doctors told me that the greater risk was that I could loose my voice forever. I was hit on the most beautiful thing in my life. That was a challenge that I had to go through.

I counted the days and the hours before the operation. For a strange "coincidence" I started receiving all sorts of information about

Reiki, what a fascinating name, I began to buy books and read information about it on the internet.

I once went to a dinner with other artists and a famous Neapolitan singer who felt my uneasiness and the suffering I had within and with a much natural gesture, put his hands on my throat. I felt such a heat. I asked him what he was doing, and he said, I am giving you love energy, it is Reiki. You can imagine my surprise.

That same evening he gave me a book to read, "The Celestine Prophecy," and from then on, I started thinking that coincidences are only in people's mind. There are no such things as coincidences.

It came the day of surgery, it was a total Thyroidectomy. I surrender myself to the hands of God.

There was more darkness around me. I was completely mute. I did not speak anymore; I did not produce any sound. I was deprived of strength and my singing career.

One vocal cord was completely paralyzed.

I was at home, in bed, and could not move. Somebody came to visit me, he gave me a brochure of a Reiki Master, the same of the Neapolitan singer that I had met at that dinner. Another coincidence? I did not think so.

I called the person and asked my husband to talk for me, we asked the Reiki Master about her next seminar.

A few weeks before taking the course, some changes were already occurring inside me. I felt some vibrations in my throat.

My husband and I went to see the doctor, and to our great surprise my vocal cord had started to vibrate again.

Which message did I take from all this? Was this my mission? My voice to give to others like a love gift.

After that seminary a new world opened for me. I began to see colors, I started wearing them, since then I only had worn black. I felt the need to color my life and to communicate to others the beauty of the simple things, like a sincere smile. My voice was changing, for the better, deeper, more intense, and straight to the hearts of the ones who listened.

A few years went by, I felt the need to continue studying Reiki, and I had to meet another Master. My intuition was right, I met my comet, the one that would have taken me by hand and let me fly again.

The rainbow has entered within me and all the unconditional love that has been donated from my great Master.
I am now here, writing all this for you dear reader, to show you that Reiki is only love energy and nothing more. As Gaetano says, listening to my voice today, transforms people's life, helps them heal their hearts. I am following my mission with great respect, honour, and love for everyone.

"We can do no great things,
We can only do small things
With great Love"

Mother Teresa

Gaetano Vivo

OPEN YOUR HEART WITH REIKI

Reiki is an ancient form of energy healing that is becoming known throughout the world as a source of unconditional love, harmony, and beauty for the Earth and its people. As we move into the new millennium, more and more of us are longing for direct experience of the spiritual realm. We look over our shoulders for angels; we turn to mediums and psychics to put us in contact with beings that are no longer, or have never been in body; we search the skies for evidence of extra-terrestrials. Our culture abounds with movies, books, documentaries and workshops on the topics of Energy Healing, Holistic Medicine and all aspects of Spirituality. In fact, the Energy has always been available to us but most of us are only now ready to embrace it. The timing of this phenomenon is not a coincidence. As our infatuation with materialism wears thin, we are opening to the possibility of connecting with higher energies to promote healing and well being. Reiki is about what is happening NOW. I teach Reiki in the tradition of my own teachers, in the line of Dr. Mikao Usui and Master Hawayo Takata. It is my goal to channel the power and beauty of Reiki into all those seeking the harmony of direct connection with universal energy for the purpose of healing.

The second part of this book is intended as a guide and reference book for all people who search for truth and harmony on our beautiful planet. It is especially meant for those who are explorers by nature, for those who are seeking light, for those who are questioning the meaning of everything in existence and for those who refuse to stand still, choosing instead, to follow the longing of their hearts. To you I say, open your hearts to the vibrations and energies of the universe and beyond. The future of Earth and all of its beings is being created now. Let those of us still in body embrace the beings of pure spirit, and, through our connection, help the healing energy of the universe flow into our future, as sacred rivers flow through the mountain passes bringing abundance to all the land.

REI UNIVERSAL ENERGY

KI LIFE FORCE

REI = The Higher Source that controls the Universe, its creation and movements. Rei is a part of everything: infinite in nature and all knowing. It acts as a source of guidance in times of need. Rei is also called God, or other names, depending on the culture.

KI = the energy that radiates from and nourishes all living things. It is essentially the life force itself, which makes up the aura. We receive Ki from food, sunshine, and the air we breathe and sleep. It is equivalent to the Chi for the Chinese, Prana for the Hindus, Baraka for the Muslims and Orenda for the Iroquois Indians and has other forms. The flow of Ki provides the healthy condition of the body. Obstructions to this flow can lead to illness.

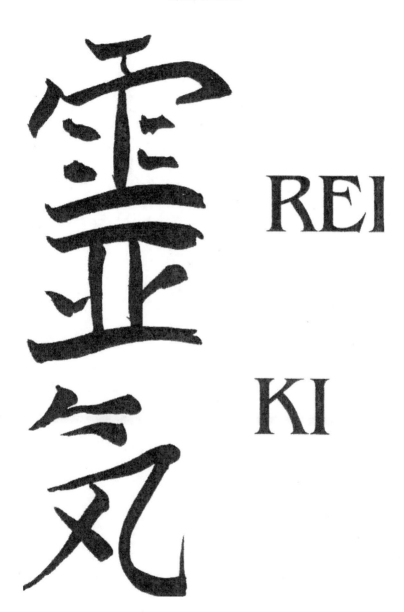

REI

KI

REIKI PRINCIPLES

JUST FOR TODAY,
DO NOT WORRY.

JUST FOR TODAY,
DO NOT ANGER

HONOR YOUR PARENTS,
TEACHERS AND ELDERS

EARN YOUR MONEY
HONESTLY

SHOW GRATITUDE TO
EVERY LIVING THING

A REIKI MASTER-TEACHER

I become a Reiki Master in Sedona, Arizona. I had always been very attracted to that town ever since I had visited it years before. I knew that something of an important meaning in my life would happen there. So it did.

I met my teacher Shalinda in June 1995, when I had gone to Sedona with some friends the first time. I heard that she was offering Reiki seminars, so I sought her out. The moment I looked into her eyes, I felt a strong connection with her. I knew that she would be my Reiki Master-Teacher.

I had been looking for something that would give greater meaning to my existence. Becoming a Reiki Master fulfilled that desire. My life has been completely transformed and enriched fully since I began my training. With Reiki, I can help people who are suffering. That is the best reward one can experience, the best success of all. It is the success of the heart, of one's life on Earth.

A true Reiki Master has to be a compassionate individual willing to change his or her own life FIRST before helping transform other people's lives. Thus, one should choose a Reiki Master with an open heart, compassion, and unconditional love.

Reiki is my passion, my life, my belief. Reiki gives me the possibility of reaching into new dimensions and parallel worlds where human eyes and perceptions alone cannot extend. Reiki is the healing form rediscovered at the beginning of the 20th century during human attempts to save the Earth. This lost healing art offers humanity a tool that can be used around the world, to shape and change human consciousness.

The world is going through many changes on many vibrational levels, as more and more we desire to be part of the healing process. There will continue to be a change in the way we think, and a change in the way we pursue our goals. We are a part of a vast reality, which seems to be evolving in ways that will affect all life, as we know it. These changes are a part of a big transformation that is happening even as we speak.

Change is the nature of all existence. People change as they grow and learn; once thriving businesses fail; banks go bankrupt; computers crash and people are afraid of the years to come. All change has to do with universal vibrations of energy originating from an unknown source. It is a higher power source, flowing to us from seemingly new dimensions and, often, new perspectives.

We are entering the Next Age. Let us do so with open hearts.

Reiki is an important part of these changes. Reiki is the way of healing for the next age. It is the healing of the future. It is one of the healing modalities that together with the use of colors, sounds and angelic energies, will allow us to survive and live more serenely in the next age.

The healing power of Reiki has been on our planet for many years. In fact, we think that it is the same healing energy Jesus channeled for His own miracles. It is a simple technique that everyone can easily learn. It is my purpose as a Reiki Master-Teacher to help others learn to open their hearts with Reiki and thus open the hearts of all society to a tranquil, loving way of life.

EARLY HISTORY AND ORAL TRADITION

The origins of the power of Reiki are as old as time. Reiki is a form of healing energy that is at the heart of the universe and of all living things. Regardless of how we, as individuals or cultures, attempt to explain the origins and nature of the planets, the universes or existence itself, we always come back to the same force, life-giving and sustaining energy. This is Reiki.

In attempting to document the history of the Reiki Healing that we know today, we can look back to the traditions established by the Buddha in India such as Gautama Siddhartha, 620-543 B.C. and to Jesus. Reiki was ancient even then. According to tradition and oral history, both of these great healers channeled pure energy through their own bodies in order to spontaneously heal suffering humanity. They also shared the same practices of fasting, meditating, and teaching through example.

It is in the line of these great teachers and healers that the historical practice of Reiki began. In the mid-1800s, Mikao Usui is said to have been associated with both the Doshisha University in Kyoto, Japan, and with the Christian ministry. Whether or not these historical alliances are fact, we know that Usui began a 10-year quest to enable him to generate the kind of healing techniques said to have been used by both the Buddha and Jesus. It is the story of the fulfillment of his quest that forms the historical origin of the Reiki that is practiced worldwide today.

Much of the information on healing was handed down orally. If a Master did not think that his students were ready, the knowledge would not be passed onwards and was often lost. Any written material on Tantric Buddhism (a form of Buddhism that included spiritual healing of mind, emotions and body) does not offer clear explanations on the Path to Enlightenment. The Tibetan Tantra Lotus Sutra, a text written in the 2nd-1st century B.C. provides the symbol formula for the Reiki technique.

DR. MIKAO USUI

The rediscovery and revival of Reiki are traditionally credited to Dr. Mikao Usui. Two different versions of his early life as a monk provide information about his identity. The first one regards him as a Christian monk, Dean of a small Christian University in Kyoto, Japan. The second one refers to him as a Buddhist Monk in Kyoto. He was born in 1865 and died in 1926. It is said that while serving as Dean of the University in Kyoto, Usui was asked by his students to demonstrate the healing method used by Jesus. He was unable to do this and began his quest to understand and learn to practice this healing skill.

During his quest, Usui sought answers to his questions about this wonderful healing ability from Christian authorities in Japan. However, when he did not receive the answers he sought, he continued his search through the study of Buddhism, since the Buddha had also practiced miraculous healing. Buddhist monks told Usui that only by studying and following Buddhist teachings could he approached spiritual healing, as the ancient healing methods had been lost.

Some sources say that Usui then traveled to the United States where he attended the University of Chicago Divinity School and studied philosophy and religion, ultimately obtaining a doctorate in Theology. He also learned to read Sanskrit, the ancient language used in Tibet and India, but his questions remained largely unanswered. In Diane Stein's, book Essential Reiki: A Complete Guide to an Ancient Healing Art, she notes that in her investigation into the history of Reiki she consulted the work of Reiki Master William Rand. According to Rand, no records to document Usui's attendance at Doshisha University as either student or principal, and no records to support the notion that Usui ever attended the University of Chicago, could be found. This discovery has led to suggestions that the Christian aspects of the story were perhaps introduced later to make Reiki more acceptable to the Christian people in the world.

Both theories of Usui's early life merge, however, when he is located in a Zen Buddhist monastery in Kyoto. Here Usui began to study Japanese, Chinese Sutras and ancient teachings of Tibet. The texts written in Sanskrit described the Reiki healing procedures and symbols, but there was no information on how to initiate the energy. According to the great Reiki Master-Teacher Hawayo Takata, the texts had been written some 2,500 years previously and had been deliberately written obscurely to protect the knowledge from misuse. It was left to Usui to interpret this newly found information. To prepare himself, he traveled to the temple on the holy mountain of Mt. Kuriyama, founded by Buddhist Priest Gantei in the year 770 B.C., to fast and meditate, alone, for 21 days. There he hoped to reach the level of consciousness described in Sanskrit texts.

It is said that Usui gathered 21 stones and placed them in front of him, with the idea that he would throw away one stone each day to count the days of his fast. It was during the last morning that he saw a ball of light on the horizon coming towards him at great speed. His first instinct was to run, but he decided to accept what was coming, and allowed the light to strike him in the center of the forehead. As it struck him, he saw rainbow-colored bubbles and the same symbols in the Tibetan writings he had studied. As he thought about the symbols, he received an attunement to each symbol and information for its use in healing.

Usui left Mt. Kuriyama with the knowledge that he now could heal as the Buddha and Jesus had done. Four miracles followed in the wake of Usui's revelations. First, Usui healed his stubbed toe while he was coming down from Mt. Kuriyama. Second, he was able to eat normally after fasting for the 21 days. Third, he healed a toothache and finally he healed the director of his monastery, who had been bedridden with an acute attack of arthritis. These miracles were signs and proof that Usui had attained the power of healing without depleting his own energy. The system of Reiki we use today evolved from the knowledge and healing practices of Mikao Usui and is called the Usui System of Natural Healing or Usui Shiki Ryoho.

Wanting to use the healing energy of Reiki to help others, Usui ventured into the slums of Kyoto. For seven years, he lived there with the beggars, helping them out of poverty and asking them to start a new life. Later he began to notice familiar faces returning, saying that life was too difficult away from the slums and that it was easier to beg. This discouraged Usui so much that he returned to the monastery. The beggars did not understand the value of the healing given, he thought, perhaps because it had been given to them; they had not paid for it. They were unwilling to take on their own responsibility in the healing process, and they focused on it primarily as a physical healing.

It was during this period that Usui received the five Spiritual Principles of Reiki that balance the physical and spiritual aspects of Reiki healing and guide all students and Masters of Reiki today. "For today only: do not anger, worry not. Do your work with appreciation. Be kind to all people. In the morning and at night, with hands held in prayer, think this in your mind, chant this with your mouth." By focusing on the spiritual level of healing, a rising of consciousness occurred in both the healer and the patient. Thus, an exchange of vital energy could take place. Hence was born the understanding of the dual responsibilities of both the healer and the healed.

Following his disappointing experience in Kyoto, Usui became a pilgrim, traveling throughout Japan, from village to village. In each village, he would stand in the streets, holding a lighted torch. When asked why he did this, he would answer that he was looking for the few interested in improving themselves and longing to be healed. Desire for healing alone was not sufficient in the eyes of Usui. It must be accompanied by a sincere desire for a change of life.

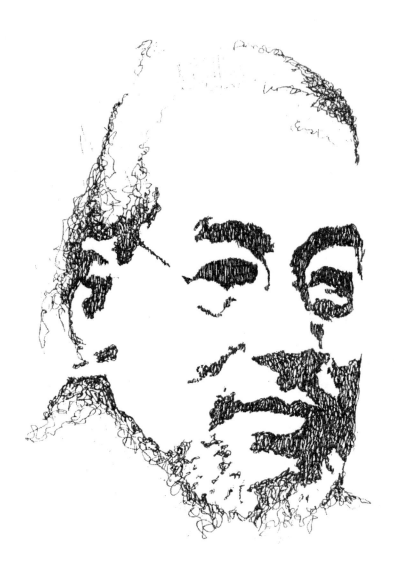

CHUJIRO HAYASHI

During his travels, Usui met Chujiro Hayashi, a retired naval officer who was impressed with Usui's sincerity. Hayashi began traveling with Usui and assisted with his lecturing. In 1925, Hayashi received his Reiki Master training from Usui and became his successor. By the time of his death in 1926, Mikao Usui had initiated 16 Reiki Masters, although sources only name Chujiro Hayashi.

Hayashi opened a clinic in Tokyo and trained teams of both male and female practitioners who worked in groups to provide healing. He also went to the homes of those unable to come to the clinic. It is to this Shina No Machi clinic that Hawayo Takata traveled from Hawaii to visit in 1935, seeking to be healed by the great Master-Teacher. It is also believed that Hayashi developed the use of the specific hand positions and the system of three degrees of training, each with its own attunement process.

HAWAYO TAKATA

In 1935, a woman named Hawayo Takata came from Hawaii to Chujiro Hayashi's clinic in Tokyo to receive healing for severe abdominal pain. She had been diagnosed with "a tumor, gallstones, appendicitis and asthma." The asthmatic condition put her at additional risk to undergo anesthesia. Some say she heard a voice telling her the surgery was not necessary. Other sources say she listened to her intuition. In any case, she had heard of Reiki treatments and, instead of undergoing surgery for her abdominal pain, she attended Hayashi's clinic. Impressed with the similarity of the hospital's diagnosis and the diagnosis given her at the clinic, she decided to try Reiki. After four months of Reiki treatment, she was completely healed.

After her healing, Takata wanted to be trained in Reiki. She had been born and raised in Hawaii by parents who were Japanese immigrants. Initially Hayashi refused her Reiki training because she was a foreigner. Hayashi wanted to keep Reiki in Japan. On the request of a Maeda Hospital surgeon, however, Hayashi finally agreed. Takata received her First Degree Reiki in 1936. She worked at Hayashi's clinic for one year, then took her Second Degree Reiki, and went back to Hawaii where she opened her own clinic.

In 1938, Chujiro Hayashi went to Hawaii to lecture and promote Reiki, and while he was there Takata received her Reiki Master training from her Master-Teacher. Following in the steps of Usui and remembering Hayashi's suggestion, Takata always charged for her Reiki treatments. Later, when she began training Reiki masters, she charged a large fee for the training. This high fee for training was not part of Usui's system but was initiated by Takata in an effort to establish Reiki as a respected field of healing.

In 1941, Hayashi summoned Takata to Japan. With war eminent, Hayashi had been drafted and he knew he would be called to duty and would be called on to perform actions that went against his spiritual development. He knew that he could not succumb to the pressure to take a human life. Fearing that Reiki would be lost to the world once more if Japan entered the war, he passed the Reiki leadership on to Takata. Hayashi decided to end his own life rather than being forced to kill others. On May 10, 1941, observed by students and family, Hayashi stopped his heart by psychic means.

The knowledge and healing practice of Reiki continued through Takata, who spread the teaching to other parts of the world. During the last 10 years of her life, Takata trained 22 Reiki Masters. She died in 1980.

Since Hawayo Takata's death, there have been many changes in the teaching of Reiki. New branches of Reiki have evolved, and new techniques have been developed. Phyllis Furumoto, Takata's granddaughter, has been named her successor and considered by many to be the Reiki Grand Master. However, Barbara Weber Ray is recognized as Grand Master by the American Reiki Association. Reiki Outreach International, founded by another of Takata's 22 Masters, Mary McFadden, considers all Reiki Masters to be equal.

During World War II, Reiki practice did indeed disappear in Japan. Thanks to Hayashi's vision and willingness to train a "foreigner," Takata, as a Reiki Master, helped the healing practice of Reiki survive the war and become known in other parts of the world. Today more and more people are learning and teaching Reiki, spreading the healing power of universal love.

Although I respect and honor the different Reiki Associations all over the world, I consider myself an independent Reiki Master.

Following are the 22 Reiki Masters who were initiated by Hawayo Takata:

1. George Araki
2. Dorothy Baba
3. Ursula Baylow

4. Rick Bockner
5. Barbara Brown
6. Fran Brown
7. Patricia Ewing
8. Phyllis Furumoto
9. Beth Gray
10. John Gray
11. Iris Ishikuro
12. Harry Kubai
13. Ethel Lombardi
14. Barbara McCullough
15. Mary McFadden
16. Paul Mitchell
17. Bethel Phaigh
18. Barbara Ray
19. Virginia Samdhal
20. Shimobu Saito
21. Seij Takimori
22. Wanja Twan

WHAT IS REIKI?

The laying of hands on the human body is not a new idea. If pain is experienced, or children injure themselves, the first thing we are inclined to do is to put our hands on the affected area, to "make it better." Human touch provides warmth and feelings of caring and love. Many kinds of therapies incorporate touch as part of the healing process.

Healing is not solely the removal of the physiological symptoms, as is commonly thought. Reiki healing is a complete process and fully resolves the cause of ill health, as well as the symptoms. Through the healing process, we return to the state of alignment with our Higher Selves – our true way of being.

Reiki is a spiritually guided technique that supplies life-force energy. The Reiki practitioner receives this energy and channels it, through the hands, into the body of the client. Working in this way with the energy centers in the body, the Reiki practitioner is able to restore a sense of well being in the client.

The origin of Reiki healing is uncertain, but it has been associated with the miraculous healing techniques of Jesus and the Buddha. Developed by Buddhist monks in Tibet, Reiki has now been adopted in the western world and is used to treat a number of different ailments, both mental and physical.

Reiki is one of the greatest gifts you can receive and share with others. Reiki is universal love, compassion, harmony, and balance that instills in the recipient a sense of power and wholeness - the path to joy and happiness. The practice of Reiki is a simple technique involving the laying of the hands on the body. Its healing touch allows the restorative energy to go through the body by way of the hands of the healer who channels this pure and clear energy from a higher source that we will call the Universe.

Students of Reiki begin by channeling this powerful energy into their own spiritual and physical bodies. A good way to practice the technique is to give Reiki to the food one eats, to the water one drinks, to one's pets, to the plants in one's home, to the room one sleeps in and to the entire house. Beginning practitioners of Reiki will soon be surprised by the vibrant energy that will surround them. It is also possible to give Reiki to any medication one may take. The universe is a daily source of this vital energy. We need only learn to accept and use it for the creation of well being. The practice of Reiki healing continues to spread as more and more people discover its benefits. It is deeply relaxing; it relieves stress and other ailments that we are subjected to in our daily lives.

It is through the hands of the Reiki Healer that the patient receives the Universal Energy. It is through his/her hands that the patient's energy becomes cleared and cleansed of energy that has accumulated in the body and is in need of release. This "stuck" energy can cause physical and emotional symptoms of illness, from mild discomfort to severe pain. The Reiki treatment works by freeing the Chakras of unwanted energies. Chakras are the energy gateways into the body. There are many Chakras, but we will be taking under consideration the seven major ones.

HOW DOES REIKI WORK?

Reiki works through attunements, which are sacred rituals that only a Reiki Master can perform. These attunements connect the healer to the source of the Universal Energy for life. The connection to the source and the ability to channel the energy is further enhanced with additional attunements. The energies of the practitioner are never depleted, as the Reiki energy is channeled. The person giving Reiki experiences an increase in Ki (the energy that radiate from and nourishes all living things), which allows him/her to perform several healing sessions in succession. The beauty of Reiki is that it is always positive, always provides healing and benefits both the Practitioner and his clients.

To connect with the Reiki Energy, the receiver places the hands upon himself/herself or on others, and spontaneously channels the energy through his/her own body. Since Reiki is guided by a Higher Intelligence, the mind and experience of the practitioner does not affect the Reiki energy. The mind of the client does not affect the healing energy, whether or not he or she believes in Reiki. The energy knows where to go and what to do.

Reiki will heal the cause of a problem on whatever level it may exist - mind, body or spirit, just as the Ki in the body can also be affected by thoughts and feelings. Negative thoughts and feelings are the main cause of restrictions to the flow of Ki. This is supported by the fact that the negative attitude and beliefs are responsible for many illnesses in the western world. Reiki bypasses the conscious mind and works directly with the unconscious one that is the repository of these thoughts and feelings, breaking them up and washing them away. Thus, the Ki flows freely and balances the functions of the physical body as well as restoring health.

If we think of the body as a house full of lights, the attunement process is similar to the act of turning on the electricity. The electrical switches connecting to the lights represent the Chakras or energy centers in the body. The Chakras link our physical bodies to our Higher Selves. These switches need to be tested, to ensure that there are no blockages to the flow of electricity. Occasionally they require repair. In the same way the Chakras in our body need to be balanced for the Ki to flow correctly. Once the switches (Chakras) are cleared of obstructions, the electricity itself (Reiki Energy) is able to flow freely and make the house (body) light up!

After being attuned, each individual will be in contact with the Universal Energy for life.

CHAKRAS

The physical body, the medium through which our consciousness is expressed, represents the lowest level of energy vibration. Our emotional, mental, and spiritual elements, of which we may not be aware, vibrate at higher frequencies than the physical body. Through our physical bodies we experienced physical movement, awareness of body parts and functions, touch, taste, smell, sight, hearing, and interaction with nature including earth and water elements.

Through our emotions we experience compassion, love, fear, doubt, the need for self-expression; opening ourselves up to joy and happiness. On the mental level, we use our conscious minds to think, plan, evaluate, and express ideas and articulate desires such as the desire for inner peace. The spiritual element focuses on the evolution of the soul.

Energy centers called Chakras (which means "wheel" in Sanskrit), are located in the body, and link these four different levels together. The Chakras link an organ, group of organs or a physical part of the body to higher levels of being. The flow of energy is adapted from pure spirit to physical manifestation. When the Chakras become unbalanced or blocked, various conditions can result ranging from phobias, fears, and mental ailments right through to physical pain and suffering.

There are numerous Chakras located throughout the body, and some of them correspond to pressure points and meridian points. We will concentrate on the major seven Chakras --Root, Sacral, Solar Plexus, Heart, Throat, Third Eye and Crown, located on an imaginary vertical line positioned in the center of the body, and mirrored on the back of the body at the same corresponding position. The Chakras are best described as spirals of light, radiating from the universe with the point of the spiral located at the chakra position on the body. In a healthy, balanced system, these points of energy or spiral light are said to "spin," channeling universal energy throughout our bodies, harmoniously linking our physical, emotional, mental, and spiritual selves.

The Chakras spin in different directions for males and females. For females the directions are as follows: Crown - counter-clockwise, Third Eye - clockwise, Throat - Counter-clockwise, Heart - clockwise, Solar Plexus - Counter-clockwise, Sacral - clockwise, Root - Counter-clockwise. For males the directions are the opposite.

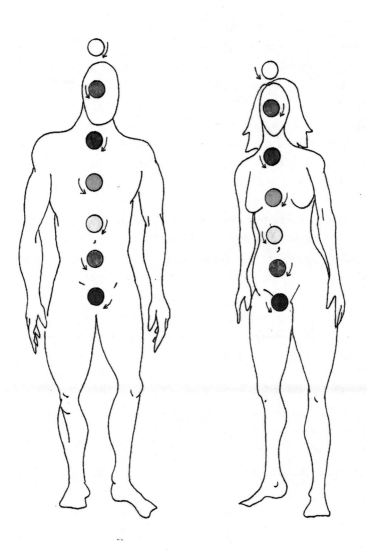

This Chakra is the source of strength and survival and is essential for proper development. The other Chakras rely upon the Root Chakra to perform properly and may be affected if it is unbalanced. The Root Chakra is situated at the base of the dorsal spine between the anus and the genitals. The color associated with the Root Chakra is Red. In the physical body, the Root Chakra is associated with the excretory system including the kidneys, bladder, intestines, bones, including the spine, also hair, nails, ejaculation, and the physical body in general.

The Root Chakra represents basic survival requirements for the body (abundance of money, food, and shelter), nutrition, security, stability, grounding, and contact with Mother Earth. The Mantra associated with this Chakra is "LAM." The representation of the Mantra is the home of Kundalini, the vital Energy (Shakti), symbolized by a sleeping snake. There are several Divinities that pertain to this Chakra: Bala Brahma, Ganesh, and Indra.

Mars is the planet analogous to the Root Chakra. Gemstones belonging to this Chakra are Agate, Red Jasper, Red Coral, Ruby, Hematite, and Obsidian. Related astrological signs include Aries, Taurus, Scorpio, and Capricorn. The parallel element is Fire, and the metal associated with the Root Chakra is Iron. Related aromas are Cedar and Cinnamon. The corresponding sense is sight.

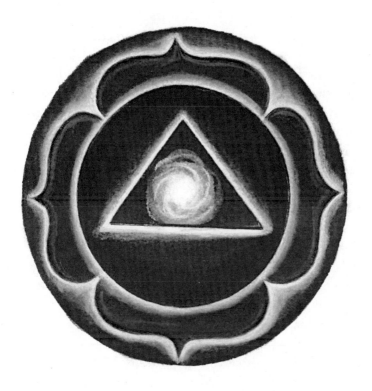

1st Chakra -- ROOT MULADHARA

The Sacral Chakra is highly influential and governs sexual and emotional energy of the body. It contains information about how experiences are felt and registered. The Sacral Chakra is located just below the navel, in the lower abdomen area between the fifth lumbar vertebra and the sacral bone. Orange is the color associated with this Chakra.

The Sacral Chakra affects everything that is fluid in the body. It regulates digestion, urine, and the sexual organs: ovaries, testicles, prostate glands, gonads, reproductive organs, lower back, bladder, kidneys, and lymphatic system.

This Chakra corresponds to relations and thoughts, how we relate to others, feelings of depression, mood swings, bodily touch, and cleanliness. The Mantra related to this Chakra is "VAM." It is symbolized by the crocodile. Vishnu is the Divinity associated with the Sacral Chakra.

The Sacral Chakra's corresponding planet is Mercury; related gemstones are Carnelian and Moonstone. Cancer, Libra, and Scorpio are the astrological signs corresponding to this Chakra. Its related element is Water, and its corresponding metal is Iron. Aromas associated with this Chakra are Ylang Ylang and Sandalwood. The corresponding sense is taste.

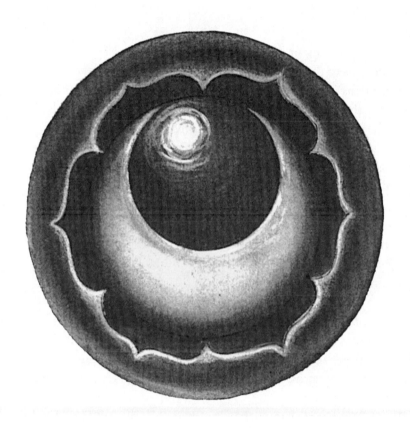

2nd Chakra -- SACRAL -- SVADHISHTHANA

The Solar Plexus, or the City of Jewels, is the ego and power centre and relates to the personality.

It contains information on the distribution of energy in the body related to personal freedom. The Solar Plexus is located at the base of the rib cage in the upper abdomen area.

The color of this Chakra is Yellow. Corresponding parts of the physical body are the digestive system: stomach, liver, gallbladder, and pancreas.

The Solar Plexus represents our hopes and fears, standing up for ourselves, how others perceive us, feelings of envy, guilt, or greed. The Mantra related to this Chakra is "RAM." Its corresponding Divinity is Braddha Rudra.

The Sun is the planet related to this Chakra. Its gemstones are Tigers'Eye, Amber, Yellow Topaz, Yellow Jasper, and Citrine. The associated astrological signs are Leo, Virgo, and Sagittarius.

Fire is the element associated with this Chakra, and its corresponding metal is Steel.

Related aromas are Lavender, Rosemary, and Bergamot. The related sense is sight.

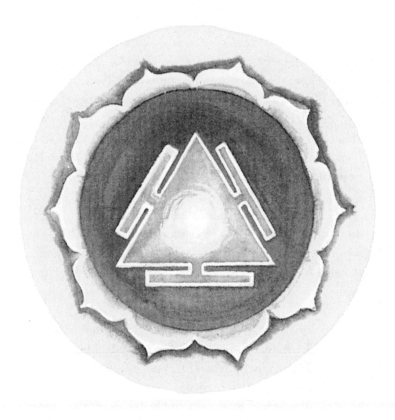

3rd Chakra -- SOLAR PLEXUS -- MANIPURA

The Heart Chakra controls self acceptance, which extends to acceptance of everybody around us. This Chakra is about unconditional love, compassion, and affinity between one's self and others. The Heart Chakra is located over the heart in the center of the body. Its associated colors are Green or Pink. In the physical body, this Chakra is related to the heart, lungs, liver, circulatory system, and pranic healing energy, with a strong influence on the vague nerve and the thymus gland.

The Heart Chakra is associated with loving ourselves, being happy with whom we are, showing love and caring for others, validation of feelings, self esteem, and detachment. The Mantra that corresponds to this Chakra is "YAM." Ishana Rudra Shiva is the corresponding Divinity.

Venus is the planet related to this Chakra; corresponding gemstones are Emerald, Green Aventurine, Rose Quartz, Malachite, Green Jade, and Pink Tourmaline. Leo and Libra are its astrological signs. The element associated with this Chakra is air, and its related metal is Silver. Rose, Rosewood, Rosemary, and Rosehips are the aromas connected with the Heart Chakra, and the corresponding sense is tactile.

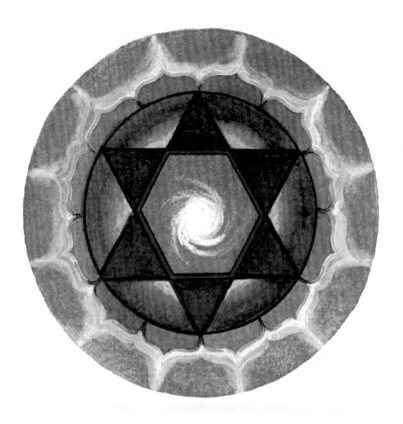

4th Chakra -- HEART-ANAHATA

Located at the base of the throat, this Chakra controls creativity, self-expression, and communication. The color associated with the Throat Chakra is Blue. In the physical body it corresponds to the throat, neck, lungs, and thyroid gland.

The Throat Chakra represents the ability to express ourselves verbally and creatively, to speak our minds, and to use language, including words and gestures. The Mantra for this Chakra is "HAM." This Chakra is associated with the Divinity, PANCHAVAKTRA SHIVA.

It is related to the planet, Jupiter, and the gemstones, Azurite, Turquoise, Lapis lazuli, Blue Agate, and Aquamarine. Astrological signs associated with this Chakra are Gemini, Taurus, and Aquarius. Its related element is Ether, and its corresponding metal is Gold. Sage, Eucalyptus, and Pine are the aromas related to the Throat Chakra. It is associated with the sense of hearing.

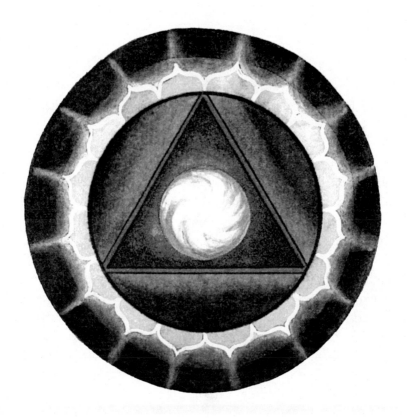

5th Chakra -- THROAT --VISHUDDHA

This Chakra is the focus of intuition, visions, and the perception of truth. Its location is in the centre of the forehead. The color associated with the Third Eye Chakra is Purple. The parts of the physical body that correspond to this Chakra are the head, pituitary gland, and nervous system.

This Chakra represents psychic abilities, awareness of guides, the will, finding our own path through life, concentration and ability to learn, dreaming, and feelings of boredom or apathy. The Mantra for this Chakra is "OM." ARDHANARISHVARA is the corresponding Divinity.

The Third Eye Chakra is associated with the planet, Saturn. Related gemstones are Amethyst and Purple Fluorite. Astrological signs associated with this Chakra are Sagittarius, Aquarius, and Pisces. Its corresponding element is Air, and its related metals are Gold and Silver. Aromas connected with this Chakra are Jasmine, Peppermint, Rosemary, and Lemongrass. Ether is the sense associated with the Third Eye Chakra.

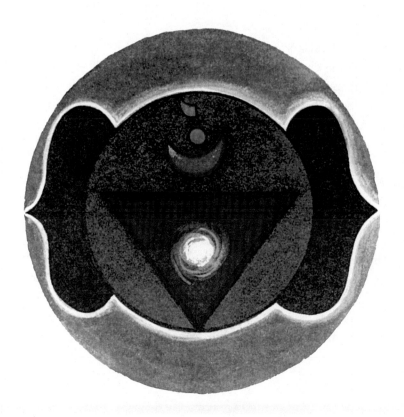

6th Chakra -- THIRD EYE --AJNA

The Crown Chakra connects us with our Higher Self, and the energy of the Universe.

The location of this Chakra is just above the head. Its color association is White, and the parts of the physical body related to this Chakra are the brain, eyes, and pineal gland.

The Crown Chakra represents spiritual states of being, ability to receive light and images, and imagination. Its Mantra is "HAOM," and the corresponding Divinity is Guru.

The planet, Moon, is closely related to this Chakra. Its corresponding gemstone is Clear Quartz and astrological signs associated with it are Capricorn, Pisces, and Cancer. Air is the element that corresponds to the Crown Chakra, and its corresponding metal is Gold. Aromas associated with this Chakra are Lavender, Neroli, Patchouli, and Rosemary. Its corresponding sense is Ether.

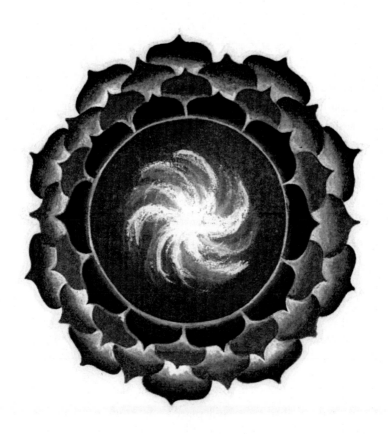

7th Chakra -- CROWN --SAHASRARA

CHAKRAS PURIFICATION MEDITATION

The practice of opening and clearing your Chakras is essential to the healing flow of Reiki Energy. This meditation will put you in touch with your seven major Chakras and help you in the process of opening them to the flow of Reiki. Sit on a comfortable chair, and place your hands on your Heart Chakra to center yourself. To call upon the Reiki Energy, begin breathing slowly in and out, rhythmically and steadily, concentrating on your breathing only. This will begin your meditation and help you to achieve a calm state of mind.

This meditation clears and cleanses the chakras, and it will give you a great sense of relaxation and inner peace.

Chakras are energetic centers which we have in the body, they need to be cleansed from cluttered energy and they must rotate in the right direction.

Sit on a comfortable chair, and place your hands on your heart chakra to centre yourself. Start breathing, slowly in and out, rhythmically and steadily. Put yourself in a calm state of mind.

Visualise all the seven chakras opening up like seven beautiful flowers

The first chakra is the Root chakra, and its colour is red. It is located approximately at the base of the spine. Visualise a gorgeous red flower opening up slowly and steadily towards the sky. In the middle of this flower there is a red wheel that rotates counter clock wise if you are a woman and clock wise if you are a man. Feel the expansion of this flower, visualise its vibrant Red colour enlarging in your root, and feel this flower filled with strong Red Light. Reflect on these feelings as you continue breathing slowly, as the Root Chakra opens to the Universal energy and we start chanting the mantra LAM and breathe deeply and slowly

After a few minutes, focus your attention on the second chakra the Sacral Chakra. Its colour is orange. It is located a few inches below the navel. Visualise a gorgeous Orange Flower opening up slowly and steadily towards the sky. In the middle of this flower there is an orange wheel that rotates clockwise if you are a woman and counter clockwise if you are a man. Feel the flower filled with strong Orange light as you continue breathing rhythmically and meditate upon the Sacral Chakra opening to the Universal Energy while chanting the mantra VAM.

Moving up your spine to the third Chakra, few inches above the navel, is the Solar Plexus chakra, its colour is yellow. Visualise a gorgeous Yellow flower opening up slowly and steadily towards the sky. In the middle of this flower there is a vibrant yellow wheel that rotates counter clockwise if you are a woman and clockwise if you are a man. Feel now the expansion of this flower, visualise this gorgeous yellow flower enlarging in the Solar Plexus and feel the flower filled with strong yellow light as it opens to Universal Energy; continue to breathe rhythmically, and focus on the feeling of the third Chakra for a few minutes and chant the Mantra RAM.

Now slowly, shift your attention to the fourth chakra the heart chakra whose colour is Green. Visualise a gorgeous Green flower opening up slowly and steadily towards the sky. In the middle of this flower there is a vibrant green wheel that rotates clockwise if you are a woman and counter clockwise if you are a man. As you breathe slowly and rhythmically, feel the expansion of this flower, visualise the gorgeous green colour expanding in the heart area, and feel that flower filled with strong green light while chanting the Mantra YAM

Visualise now the fifth chakra, the Throat, its colour is blue. Imagine a gorgeous blue flower opening up, slowly and steadily towards the sky. In the middle of this flower there is a vibrant blue wheel that rotates counter clockwise if you are a woman and clockwise if you are a man. Feel the expansion of this flower, see the gorgeous blue colour enlarging in the throat area, and feel that flower filled with strong blue light while chanting the Mantra HAM.

Moving your attention now to the centre of the forehead just above your eyes, is the Sixth chakra, the Third Eye, its colour is Purple. Visualise a gorgeous purple flower opening up slowly and steadily towards the sky. In the middle of this flower there is a purple wheel that rotates clockwise if you are a woman and counter clockwise if you are a man. Feel the expansion of this flower, sense the vibrant purple colour enlarging in the Third Eye chakra, and experience that flower filled with strong purple light while chanting OM.

Finally shift your attention on the Seventh Chakra, the Crown Chakra, its colour is White, and it is located on the top of your head. Visualise a gorgeous white flower opening up slowly and steadily towards the sky. In the middle of this flower there is a gorgeous white wheel that rotates counter clockwise if you are a woman and clockwise if you are a man. Feel the expansion of this flower, sense and see its vibrant white colour expanding in the crown area, and experience that flower filled with strong white light and chant the Mantra HAOM.

Now all of your Chakras are wide open, rotating in the right direction.

Visualise a beam of Golden light coming down from the Universe, pouring its light into your body, cleansing and clearing all the chakras one by one. At the same time, a beam of Silver light comes from Mother Earth into your root Chakra giving your body an Earthly Vibration. Feel the two beams meeting at the Solar Plexus Chakra and mixing together, giving you a sense of peace throughout the body.

Breath slowly and visualize your chakras closing one by one making sure that the wheels in the middle keep rotating in the right direction forever…

Now you can slowly open your eyes and feel around you a sense of unconditional love permeating all over you and your surroundings...

FIRST DEGREE REIKI

PERFORMING A REIKI TREATMENT

Each time you give a Reiki treatment to a relative, a friend or to a client, it is a good custom to wash your hands before you start, and at the end of each treatment. This practice washes away unwanted energy.

Have your client lie down comfortably on a treatment table. Remove all metals from your body, jewels, belt, and coins in the pocket. Ask your client to do the same. This allows a better flow of the energy from the healer into the body of the receiver. Remove your shoes and ask your client to do the same. If possible, play soothing music in the room.

Place your hands on your Heart Chakra to call upon the Universal Energy, asking for healing for that person in that time. Imagine that your heart Chakra is like a large green button. You push the button in when you want to call upon the Universal Energy. You push the button back out, when you conclude a treatment and you want to stop the flow of energy.

After you have called upon the Universal Energy, start sweeping the Aura of your client, placing your hands a few inches above his/her body. Begin at the Crown Chakra and move downward in a very slow and gentle motion. I stress that this movement must be extremely slow to avoid causing any traumas or discomfort to your client. The first sweep is done on the middle of the body, the second and the third are on the left and the right side of the body.

While caressing the Aura you will experience all sorts of sensations: coolness, warmth, tingling sensations in your hands. This will be the first interaction you have with your client's energy. Those sensations will tell you the places in the client's body that you need to work on the most. Trust these sensations and follow your intuition.

The Aura is the energy field that surrounds every living being. When you sweep the Aura, just let the energy come. Let your hands move down the body freely without any resistance. Do not concentrate too hard. Feel free to receive the energy and pass it onto the client. The energy will come and flow freely from your hands onto the Aura of your client.

Open the Chakras of your client with a circulating movement a few inches above the body, rotating your hands in the direction of the Chakra. At the end of the treatment, while the client is turned on the stomach, you will close the Chakras with the same movement circulating your hands in the opposite directions of the Chakra themselves.

It is necessary to receive attunements, to get a connection with the Reiki Energy before being able to perform a Reiki treatment.

1. Get yourself into a relaxed and meditative state of mind.

2. Try to maintain physical contact with the client.

3. When moving your hands to a new position on the person's body, move them one hand at a time to keep the connection with the energy.

5. Apply a gentle touch always when performing the hand positions.

Remember to quickly flick your fingers (Reiki Off) after each treatment.

HAND POSITIONS

A: With the person lying face up:

THE HEAD

1. Sitting behind the person who is lying on the treatment table, place your hands for at least 3   minutes on the sides of the face, with the tips of the fingers on each side of the client's chin.
2. Moving the hands, one at a time, place your hands over the client's ears.
3. Next, place your hands over the client's eyes, resting the base of the palms on the client's forehead, and crossing your thumbs. Leave the nose exposed with enough space for the person to breathe.
4. Moving your hands slowly, one at a time, place your hands on the top of their head.
5. Next, place your hands on each side of the client's head and turn it slowly to each side, carefully moving the upper

hand to the back of the head. Rotate the client's head to the original position, using the lower hand, and then move this hand to the back of the head (you are now holding the client's head in your hands).

6.   Now move one hand to the back of the client's neck, and place the other across the forehead.

Finally, keep one hand on the back of the client's neck, and move the other hand to the Heart Chakra area.

THE BODY

Place one hand on the client's Heart Chakra, the other one on the Throat Chakra a few inches above the body. A client will feel a sense of suffocation if you touch his/her throat.

7.   Place your hands on the client's shoulders.

8.   Move to the side of the person, and while standing, place your hands, palms down, across the client's upper chest area, just below the throat. The tips of the fingers on one hand should touch the inside of the wrist of the other hand.

9.   Next, place your hands on the client's upper abdomen area (base of the ribs—Solar Plexus).

10.   Finally, place your hands on the client's lower abdomen area.

OPTIONAL

Keeping one hand on the client's lower abdomen, place the person's hand that is furthest from you, on top of yours and cover it with your free hand.

Keeping one hand on the client's lower abdomen, and place your free hand on top of the person's hand which is closest to you. Place your hands on the client's hips.

THE LEGS

11. Place your hands on the client's thighs.
12. Place your hands on the client's knees.
13. Place your hands on the client's shins.
14. Next, stand or sit at the end of the table and hold the client's legs by supporting the ankles from underneath, one in each hand. While in this position, send energy through your left hand into the body, receiving it again from the client's body into the right hand. Continue to send energy to the body in this cycle.
15. Place your hands so that they are cupped over the top of the client's toes.
16. Working with one foot at a time, move one hand to the side of the client's foot and wrap it around the top part of the foot. Wrap the free hand around the center of the same foot, with the thumb pressed into the center of the sole.
17. Repeat the above step for the other foot.
18. Press each thumb in the center of each foot to complete this part of the healing session.

Now, shake your hands three times to wave the energy away.

Once you have shaken your hands:

19. Go back to the breast of your patient placing your hands few inches above the body and send Reiki energy to it. Then go on the genitals:

A: For women, form a "V" a few inches above the body (pointing towards the feet) with your hands,
B: For men, the hands are placed side by side over the genitals, a few inches above the body.

NOTE: Under the soles of the feet there are two major Chakras. It is from these Chakras that the unwanted energy passes out of the body during a Reiki treatment. That is why your patient will feel all sorts of sensations in the feet during a Reiki healing.

Now, ask your client to roll over on the stomach.

B. With the person lying face down:

THE HEAD

1. Sit behind the person lying on the treatment table, and place your hands on the back of the head.
2. Next, place your hands on the upper shoulder area.
3. Stand by the side of the person. Form a "T" at the top of the client's back (one hand across the shoulders and the other hand placed along the spine, such that the fingers touch the first hand).
4. Place your hands palms down (with the tips of the fingers on one hand touching the inside of the wrist of the other hand as before), in the middle of the back (Heart Chakra area).
5. Place your hands approximately one hand width further

down the client's back (Solar Plexus Chakra area).

6.   Form a "T" at the base of the back, with one hand across the base of the client's spine and the other resting over the buttocks, with your fingers touching your first hand.

7.   Place your hands few inches above the client's buttocks (one pointing towards the head, one towards the feet).

THE LEGS

8.   Place your hands across the back of the client's thighs.

9.   Next, place your hands on the back of the knees.

10.   Now, lace your hands across the client's calves.

11.   Support the client's ankles again, standing or sitting at the end of the table. Send energy into the body a cycle through your left hand, receiving it again through your right hand.

12.   Place your palms flat against the soles of the client's feet.

Close each of the Chakras in the opposite direction to that used to open them, starting with the Crown Chakra. (i.e., if your client is a woman, you start closing the Crown Chakra rotating your hand three times clockwise, and so on.)

Sweep the Aura once, over the middle of the body.

Hold your palms down, over the middle of the person's body and quickly close and open your hands, to stop the Reiki Energy (Reiki Off).

Cross your hands over your heart, thanking the energy and physically step back. In so doing, you exit the Aura of your client. Any vibrations that come from that person will not stay with you but will remain with the person.

The Universal Reiki Energy that we channel comes in a very pure and cleansing form. It is very powerful and washes away all the unwanted energy from the channeler first, then from the person receiving the energy. That is why I always stress that once you perform a Reiki Treatment the energy that comes through cleanses and clears the energy of the healer first. In this way the healer does not put any of his unwanted energy into the client and vice-versa.

I always teach my students to step back physically, because in that way, we virtually exit the Aura of the person we are treating in that moment. You might feel vibrations that do not belong to you while performing a treatment; those vibrations leave your body when you conclude the treatment.

Reiki treatments can be silent or not. You can talk during the treatment if you wish to do so. There are people who prefer to talk during the performance of Reiki, and there are others who prefer to just relax and maybe sleep.

Sometimes, it is necessary for the Reiki practitioner to talk to his/her clients. For instance, if they feel blockages in the Chakras, sometime it is beneficial to discuss it with the client. I have created an exercise that allows people to heal themselves with the aid of the Reiki Energy.

If you feel, for instance, that the Heart Chakra of your client is not functioning properly, put your hand on that Chakra for few minutes. Ask your client to visualize your hand to be a magnet, so that he/she can feel all the unwanted energies leaving that particular

Chakra and going into your hand.

Usually after few minutes of this exercise the client starts feeling all sorts of emotions coming up. This is a good sign. It means that the Chakra is clearing out and starting to spin again. A good way of getting the unwanted energy completely out of the body is to ask your client to inhale by their nose, and as he/she exhales through the mouth, he/she lets out all the unwanted energy. The practitioner can actually feel the energy going away from the client's feet Chakras. Ask the client to repeat this process three times. Very often, at the end of this exercise, the feet of the client become cold. It is a good practice for the Reiki healer to give or send extra Reiki Energy to the feet.

Do this exercise with all the Chakras that you feel are not functioning properly.

The Reiki healer, acting as a medium for the flow of energy, needs to be protected while performing such a treatment. It is important to place your right hand on the person's Chakra. Make sure that your left hand points downward, allowing the unwanted energy coming from the person to exit through your left hand. Consciously send this energy back into the Universe. Remember that you are only a medium for the flow of these powerful energies. Act only as a go-between for your client's energy and the Universal Energy.

Usually, blockages in the major Chakras occur because people have been subjected to emotional turmoil, anxiety, and worries for a long time. That is why we have to make sure that those little wheels rotate in the right directions all the time. When one of those wheels stops, the Chakra automatically becomes blocked and the energy stops flowing. When this happens, physical and emotional illness and pain occur.

THE REIKI BOOST

If time is restricted, the location is not suitable, or if the person is not comfortable lying down, you can perform a quick form of treatment. This includes all of the most important Reiki positions, and concentrates on the Chakras.

Make use of the time available and get yourself into a relaxed and meditative state of mind. Even a short treatment can provide wonderful results.

No contact is made with the person at any time during the Reiki Boost, and the sweeping of the Aura should be done slowly. The person should be standing or sitting in a chair.

Concentrate on the Chakra positions when sweeping over the body.
Cross your hands over your heart and call on the Universal Energy.
Sweep the Aura front and back, at the same time, with both hands.
Sweep the Aura on both sides of the body at the same time.
Place your hands over the client's Crown Chakra, and then slowly pass your hands down over both sides of the head to the Third Eye Chakra.
Move your hands down so that one is at the front of the client's Throat Chakra and the other is at the back of the his/her neck.
Sweep one hand down to the Heart Chakra, with the other hand at an equal distance from the back of the body.
Sweep down to the Solar Plexus Chakra area, front and back.
Sweep down to the Sacral Chakra area, front and back.

Sweep down to their Root Chakra, front and back.
Sweep all the way down the front and back of the legs to the ground.

Cross your hands over your heart, and thank your guides.

SELF TREATMENT

It is beneficial for you to practice Reiki on yourself as much as possible to become accustomed to the energy. You can start your morning with a Reiki treatment on yourself; it is energizing, empowering and will put your mind at peace for the day.

You can also give yourself a treatment while lying in bed or before you go to sleep at night. Working with the higher Chakras only, will give you a soothing relaxing sleep. Sometimes you will wake up with your hands still in the same Reiki positions as when you fell asleep the night before.

To perform a Reiki self-treatment, follow these steps:

Remain between 3 to 5 minutes in each hand position.
Remember to move your hands one at a time when changing to the next position.
Treat any part of the body that requires healing energy.
Sit down and cross your hands over your heart to connect with the Reiki Energy.

1.   Place your hands on the sides of your face for at least 3
        minutes.
2.   Place your hands over your ears.
3.   Place your hands over your eyes.
4.   Place one hand across your forehead, the other across the
        back of your neck.
5.   Place both hands on the back of your head, with the base
        of the palms resting at the back of the neck, and cross
        the thumbs. Place both hands horizontally, one above the

other, at the back of the head.

6.   Now place your hands around your neck.

7.   Next, place your hands on the upper chest.

8.   Now move your hands to the breast area.

9.   Place your hands on the Solar Plexus area.

10.   Now place your hands on the lower abdomen area.

11.   Slowly move your hands to the genitals.

12.   Then place your hands on your thighs.

13.   Place your hands on your knees.

14.   Keep your right hand on your right knee and rest this leg across the thigh of the left leg. With the free hand, hold the ankle of the right leg. You should now be holding the knee and the ankle of the right leg, while sitting in an upright position.

15.   Now, move your hands so that one is on the right ankle and the other hand is wrapped around the middle of the right foot.

16.   Next, place one hand on the sole of the right foot and the wrap the other hand around the top of the foot. Repeat the above 3 steps for the left leg.

17.   Place your hands on the lower back around the kidney area.

Finally, cross your hands over your heart and thank your Reiki guides.

SECOND DEGREE REIKI

A major portion of Second Degree Reiki consists of a set of three Symbols with a vibration of the highest spiritual implication when utilized properly: CHO KU REI (pronounced Cho Koo Ray), SEI HE KI (pronounced Say Hey Key) and HON SHA ZE SHO NEN (pronounced Hon Sha Zoo Sho Nen). These three Symbols, together with other Reiki Master symbols, were the same ones that Mikao Usui received on Mt. Kuriyama during his 21-day period of fasting and meditation. Once again, both the literal meanings and applications as well as the illustrations of the three Symbols are presented here in an effort to be true to the dual nature of Reiki teaching and practice, as both spiritual and physical healing. The energy that makes the Symbols active can only be received from a Reiki Master; otherwise the Symbols by themselves have no value. In order to receive the Symbols, students must be prepared for the four attunements,

When the practitioner uses the Symbols in healing practice, whether it is of body, mind, or spirit, they have to be visualized in violet light, at the same time as they are drawn over the body of the client. Every time you apply a different Symbol to the client, different forces are made active. The degree of the power of activation is very much dependent on the accuracy of the drawing of the Symbol.

Each of the Reiki II Symbols should be memorized, and can be drawn in different ways. For example, with the palm of the hand and with the fingers together, or with the palm of the hand and with the fingers apart, or by using the thumb together with the first two fingers all closed together. The Symbols are usually illustrated

with direction arrows, which show how they should be drawn.
Some students who take Reiki II have a recollection of the Symbols,
as they are placed in the Aura during the Reiki I attunement. Before
the Symbols are seen visually in Reiki II, they are already channeled
with Reiki Energy through the hands. Once a Reiki Master attunes
you to the Symbols and their use, this constitutes a sacred verbal
agreement which is not to be revealed. You owe it to yourself and
your teacher to keep the sacredness of the Symbols intact.

Gaetano Vivo

REIKI II SYMBOLS

At the time of Mrs. Takata, the symbols had to remain covert and
no one other than a Reiki Master could look at them. Nowadays
things have changed and since the vibration of Earth has accelerated,
there is no more time for hidden teachings. Since the publication of
Diane Stein's book, Essential Reiki, the Reiki Symbols no longer
remain a secret. Her rationale in publishing the Symbols was that
in today's fast-paced world, we learn more from books than from
long periods of time sequestered with Master Teachers. Therefore,
to make Reiki healing more accessible to all who choose to study
and practice it, she published the Reiki Symbols. I, also, have chosen
to publish the Reiki Symbols in the belief that the more we open
our hearts towards the healing power of Reiki, the better it is for
more people to understand and appreciate the healing work that we
are carrying out.

I understand that the Japanese culture is a very secretive one. When
the symbols were channeled they could have been shown only to the
diligent students. A century has gone by, and changes are happening
so rapidly that there is no time for us to still hide things away.
Everything has to be in the open now.

There are Reiki Masters nowadays who have chosen to make the
Symbols available to everybody. If you are not attuned to Reiki II
you will not be able to perceive the energy of the Symbols. When
a Reiki Master has opened your channels for that specific energy,
then the right energy will work for you and others.

I have decided to show the Symbols in my book for those people
who teach Reiki and for the learners who need to practice how to

draw them.

I will always maintain the theory that Reiki is love energy and should be taught to as many people possible, and especially to the young people, who are our future. Reiki is an exchange of energy and we are energy, so there will be always a shift of energy when you give or receive Reiki, or when you are attuned to this vibrant energy.

CHO KU REI

Cho Ku Rei (pronounced Cho Koo Ray) is a Tibetan Symbol with a mixture of Indian Sanskrit. This Symbol in Reiki is known as the "light switch" and is used to direct and focus power. The spiral shape represents a conch shell, symbolizing the calling to the heavens. Spirals always represent Universal Energy. By visualizing the Cho Ku Rei Symbol, your ability to access the Reiki Energy is increased many times. The Reiki is focused in one area by calling all the Universal Energy into the healing. This symbol has a masculine energy.

Cho Ku Rei increases the healing power when drawn on certain parts of the body, or used in conjunction with other Reiki Symbols.

Cho Ku Rei, can be used to increase the power of a room, or to energize a crystal, or water. Draw the Cho Ku Rei symbol three times in the middle of a room. A therapy room energized with the Cho Ku Rei is a great gift to your clients.

The Symbol has to be drawn clockwise. The Symbol should be drawn three times and the words "Cho Ku Rei" should be said mentally, each time that the Symbol is drawn. Use the Symbol at any time during a healing session.

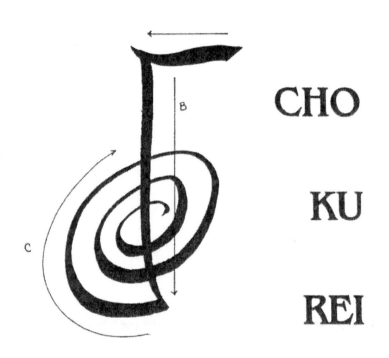

CHO

KU

REI

A Swirl of light, Power increase

SEI HE KI

Sei He Ki (pronounced Say Hey Key) is a Japanese Symbol. It is used to align the body, balancing the upper four Chakras at the emotional level. A large number of physical ailments and diseases have an emotional cause. If emotional pain and traumas are not released, or feelings are not expressed, these can manifest as a physical illness. Healing the disease also means healing the emotions with which it is associated. This symbol has a feminine energy.

When giving a Reiki Treatment, you can draw the Sei He Ki Symbol on the body of the person three times. Doing so helps their Chakras to start working and opening up, and the energy will start becoming cleared and cleansed. Reiki Energy goes to where it is needed on every level of our physical, emotional, mental and spiritual bodies. The emotional aspect is specifically addressed by using the Sei He Ki Symbol. The client reconnects with this emotional pain long enough to let it go, resulting in the clearing of the physical disease.

Sei He Ki is used for purification, and to clear unwanted energy. Place the Sei He Ki Symbol on the palm of your hand, and, with that, you can purify, clear and cleanse anything, from a room that needs clearing to a crystal or to water.

You can use the Sei He Ki Symbol in conjunction with the Cho Ku Rei Symbol. These two symbols together clear and energize, giving to your belongings a vibrant pure and crystalline energy.

For protection from lower energies, always visualize Sei He Ki around you all the time.

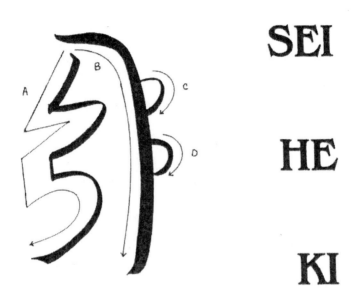

SEI

HE

KI

Chakra Balancer and connection, purification
clearing, cleansing

HON SHA ZE SHO NEN

Hon Sha Ze Sho Nen (pronounced Hon Sha Zoo Sho Nen) is a Japanese Symbol.

It is used to send absent healing, and to build a healing bridge to a person not physically present. The Symbol translates as "the Buddha in me, reaches out to the Buddha in you," or another meaning "no past, no present, no future." Hon Sha Ze Sho Nen heals the past, the present and the future in these and other lifetimes. The Hon Sha Ze Sho Nen is the Symbol that transmits Reiki energy across distance, space and time. It is the most complex of the Reiki Symbols to draw.

Using the Symbol in a healing session can change past traumas, and those changes can be brought into the present, which will practically change the future. It produces a domino effect which can only cause positive results. For almost every event in this lifetime, a past life or karmic pattern may be discovered. The Hon Sha Ze Sho Nen helps to complete and release the karma, which creates the process in the conscious mind.

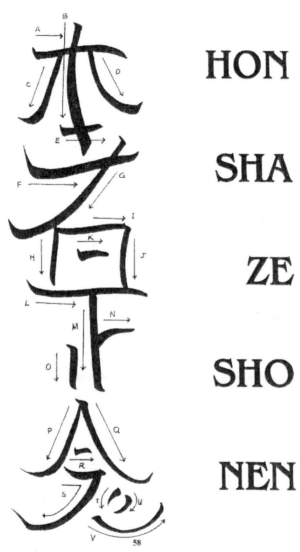

HON

SHA

ZE

SHO

NEN

Absent or Distant Reiki Symbol

ABSENT HEALING

Absent healing has the same energy and power as physically laying your hands on somebody. It is your intention to heal which is the most important consideration. Hon Sha Ze Sho Nen is the key to unlocking the door to connect to a person at a distance. Connect with the name of the person, draw the Symbol and allow the energy to flow through yourself toward your intention. Remember, Reiki is only used for the highest good, so do not become involved in the outcome of the absent healing. Learn to trust.

Start the absent healing by having before you a representation of the person to be treated. This can be a photograph, any object that reminds you of the person, a doll or teddy bear, or by visualizing him or her in your mind. Next you must have permission to perform the healing. This is part of the ethics of Reiki, and holds true for absent healing also. Follow your intuition, as you will receive an answer or message. If you are not sure of the answer, send the absent healing with the intention that it is to be accepted by the free will of the person to be healed.

In a meditative state, while holding the representation of the person in your hands, visualize the Hon Sha Ze Sho Nen in a violet light, coming out of your Third Eye and Heart Chakras. See it entering the body of the person through the Crown Chakra. I usually advise my students to visualize the Symbol leaving those two points of energy, then forming a triangle shape or a missile. Once inside the body of the recipient, the symbol explodes in thousand of vibrant fine particles going to treat the parts needing help.

During the healing, be open to what you see, and do not impose limitations on the energy. When you have finished, return to the present and forget the healing to release the energy to the person. You can nominate to send absent healing at a fixed time to repeat the session, if necessary. Absent healing can be sent in exactly the same way to yourself, a person or event in the past, to a current situation, to people you do not know and to the Planet. An old photograph or an explanation on paper of the situation or event can be held during the absent healing session.

This technique can also be used when the person is present, as in cases where placing the hands on the body is not appropriate, when the person is asleep, when there is not enough time, when touching the person would cause pain or when there is a risk of infection.

For performing self healing, take a picture of when you were little, or a picture when you experienced traumas in your childhood or adolescence, or a picture of some years ago. When you send absent Reiki healing to that picture, you will experience all sorts of emotions coming up. You will know that you are on the right path to transforming your present life.

The following meditation can be used to send energy in the past so that our present will be brighter and sunnier.

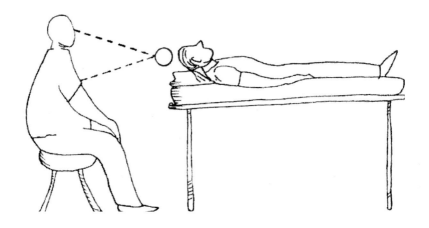

A distant Reiki treatment

KARMA PURIFICATION MEDITATION

The karma meditation will allow you to release and cleanse your Karma, slowly and with a lot of good will…

All Karmic models which we are born with come from a previous life, and growing up today on Earth, we need to feel clear energy channels and spiritually more aware.

Forget the daily worries and problems for few minutes, taking care of your self, concentrate on your body and mind.

Visualize now the seven chakras opening…..

The first chakra is the Root chakra, and its colour is red. It is located approximately at the base of the spine. Visualise a gorgeous red flower opening up slowly and steadily towards the sky, loose yourself completely into the music.
The root chakra is related to three months before birth, visualize yourself in your mother's womb three months before you were born, try to discover different sensations, try to understand where you are, and which is your path. Send energy to that situation in your past, through the first chakra, putting your hands on it. Well done.
After a few minutes, begin focusing your attention on the second chakra the Sacral Chakra whose colour is orange. It is located a few inches below the navel. Visualise a gorgeous orange flower opening up slowly and steadily towards the sky, loose yourself in the music

related to the second chakra. ------- The sacral chakra is related to your birth. See yourselves coming out of your mother's womb, explore the world around you, take a glimpse of your parents for the first time, for some of us birth has been beautiful for others more traumatic, therefore with so much love, and so much joy, send energy to this situation in the past, send energy to your birth so that you can heal situations in the present. Place your hands on the second chakra and feel the sensations you are experiencing riberthing.

Moving up your spine to the third Chakra, few inches above the navel, is the Solar Plexus whose colour is yellow. Visualise a gorgeous yellow flower opening up slowly and steadily towards the sky, loose yourself completely to the music related to the Solar plexus chakra. This chakra is connected with your childhood, when the child goes from the spiritual world to a material one, approaching the social events of life, society, school...the child can be traumatized during this passage, to help him going through these changes, place your hands on the third chakra and send energy to that situation. Breathe deeply and slowly...

Slowly, shift your attention to the fourth chakra the heart chakra its colour is Green. Visualise a gorgeous Green flower opening up slowly and steadily towards the sky. Abandon yourself to the energy of the music related to this chakra, the heart chakra is the house of your emotions, your passions, and it is related to your adolescence, place your hands on the heart chakra and send energy into the past, to your emotional life, so that you can heal situations of that time, send thoughts of love and forgive situations and people related to that period of your life. And keep breathing....
Visualise now the fifth chakra, the Throat chakra, its colour is blue.

Imagine a gorgeous blue flower opening up, slowly and steadily towards the sky. The throat chakra is related to your present, the expression of creativity, communication with yourselves and others, to heal the way we communicate love, affection and to forgive. Give universal energy to the throat chakra and send love thoughts--------
- forgiving situations and people related to your daily world. Loose yourself in the music and feel the vibrations of the throat chakra rising to a higher frequency…and keep breathing…

Move your attention now to the centre of the forehead just above your eyes, this is the Sixth chakra, the Third Eye, and its colour is Purple. Visualise a gorgeous purple flower opening up slowly and steadily towards the sky------------ lose yourself in the music ----
------this will get you a vision of a past life, so that you can heal karmic issues related to a specific past life, send loving energy to that life, may be you will see an image, a flower, a shape, or may be something you have never seen before, doing that loose yourself in the vibrations that the music gives you and keep breathing slowly and deeply..

Finally shift your attention on the Seventh Chakra, the Crown Chakra, its colour is White, and it is located on the top of your head. Visualise a gorgeous white flower opening up slowly and steadily towards the sky. The seventh chakra is related to your future, abandon yourself completely to the music, sending energy to future events in your life, you will get a total relaxation and great sense of well being.

The seven chakras now, vibrate at a very high frequency , with the aid of the music, you will feel a total sense of wellbeing so that you can clean and purify your karma, slowly and gradually, walking the spiritual path, feeling at peace, and ready to give universal love to yourselves.

Breathe slowly and visualize your chakras closing one by one…

You can now slowly open your eyes and feel around you a sense of unconditional love permeating all over you and your surroundings.

THE TEACHINGS OF REIKI

The teaching of Reiki I & II level takes 16 hours per level.

All the Reiki levels consist of 4 attunements or initiations. These are sacred rituals that only a Reiki Master can perform. It is during these rituals that the Reiki Master opens each student's channels so that they can start receiving the Universal Energy.

The Reiki I level consists of:

The History of Reiki
The Reiki Principles
Performing a Reiki treatment
Preparation for attunement
Meditation before the attunements
Four attunements per person, if the course is taught in two days you can give people two attunements per day.
Closing meditation
How to perform a self treatment
Reiki Boost
Diploma ceremony

The Reiki II Level consists of:

Symbols
Absent Reiki Healing
Using Symbols during Treatments
Preparation for the four Attunements of Reiki II
Four attunements per person, if the course is taught in two days you can give people two attunements per day

Gaetano Vivo

Chakra Spinning
Diploma ceremony

THIRD DEGREE REIKI

The teachings of Reiki III are deep and interesting at the same time. I teach Reiki I and II in one weekend or in two separate weekends. The teaching of Reiki III, however, requires more than a weekend to learn. I teach Reiki III over the course of three years. I have chosen to do so because the students appreciate and begin to feel their Mastership, and slowly come to understand that practicing and teaching Reiki is what they want to do with their lives.

One of the advantages of studying Reiki III for three years are that students get to know their Master better as a role model and achieve a certain bond with the Master that never dies. Becoming a Reiki Master can be a transforming experience, changing your life forever.

Students learn how to deal with all sorts of issues. I, some times, take my students with me if there is a case that needs to be seen in a group situation. In this way, students can observe the Master delivering Reiki to a person who is an invalid or handicapped. Attending Reiki healings of such disorders in a group with their Master is a valuable lesson for Reiki III students.

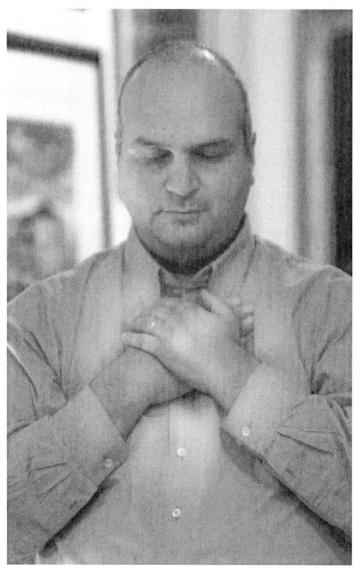

HANDS ON THE HEART CHAKRA TO CENTER YOURSELF

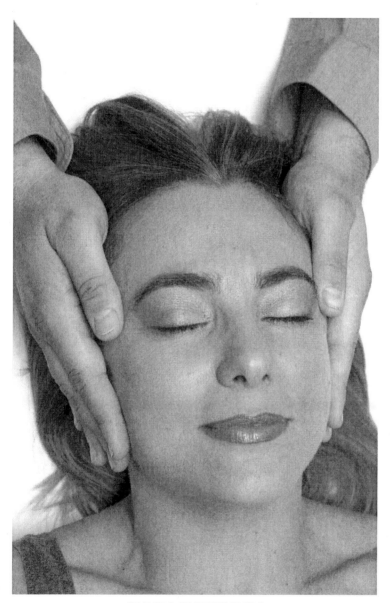

HANDS ON THE EARS

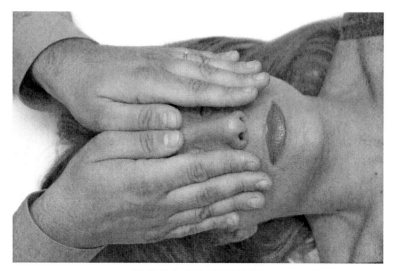

HANDS ON THE EYES

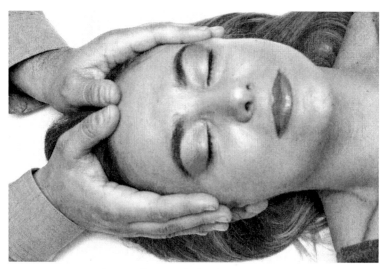

HANDS ON THE CROWN CHAKRA

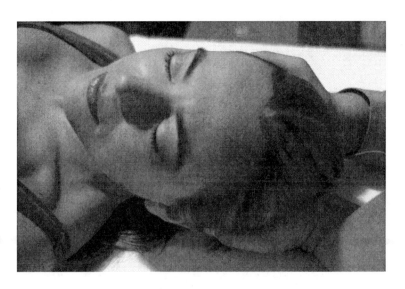

HANDS UNDER THE HEAD

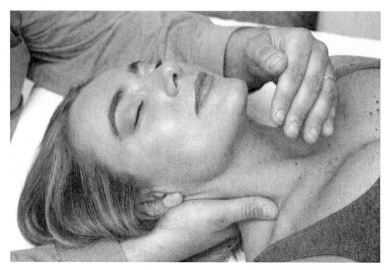

HANDS ON THE THROAT

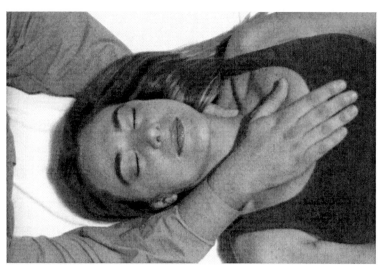

ONE HAND ON THE HEART CHAKRA AND ONE ON THE NECK

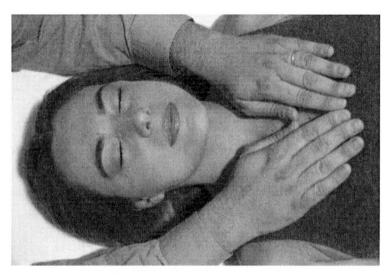

HANDS ON THE HEART CHAKRA

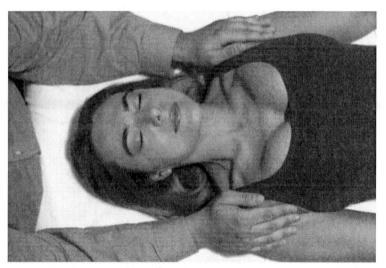

HANDS ON ARMS AND SHOULDERS

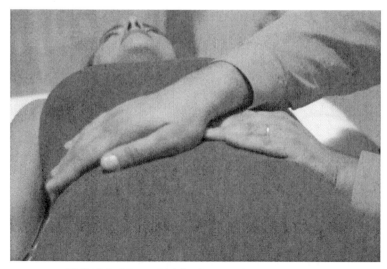

HANDS ON THE SOLAR PLEXUS CHAKRA

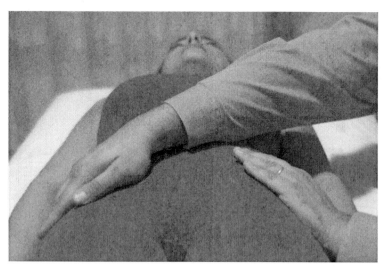

HANDS ON THE SACRAL CHAKRA

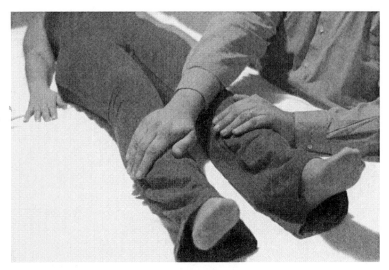

HANDS ON THE KNEES

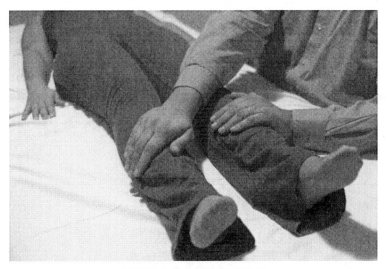

HANDS ON THE SHINS

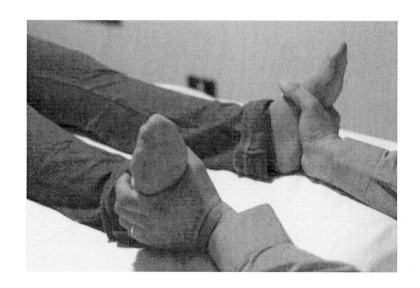

HANDS UNDER THE FEET

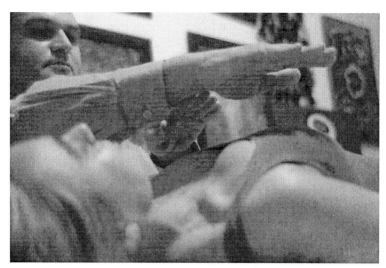

DISTANT HANDS ON THE BREAST

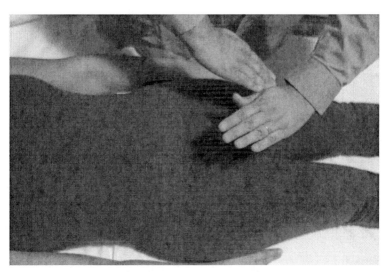

DISTANT HANDS ON THE ROOT CHAKRA

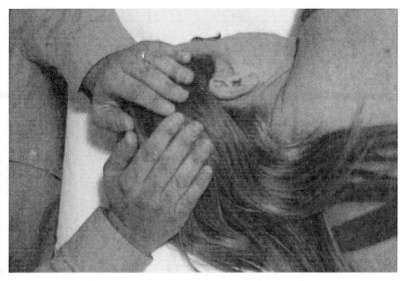

HANDS ON THE CROWN CHAKRA

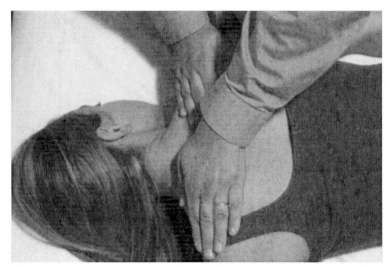

HANDS ON THE SHOULDERS

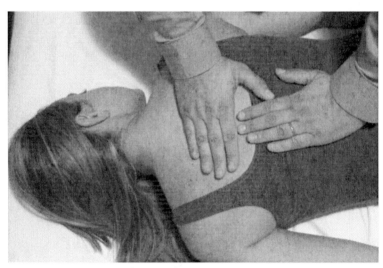

T POSITION ON THE BACK BALANCING THE UPPER CHAKRAS

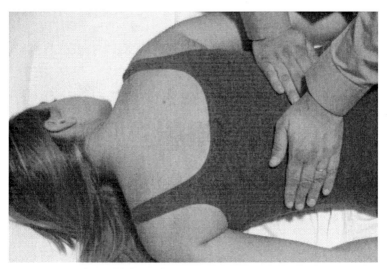

HANDS ON THE LOWER BACK AND KIDNEYS

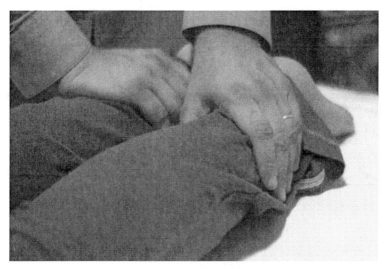

HANDS ON THE CALVES

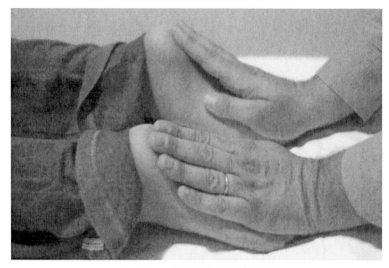

HANDS UNDER THE FEET

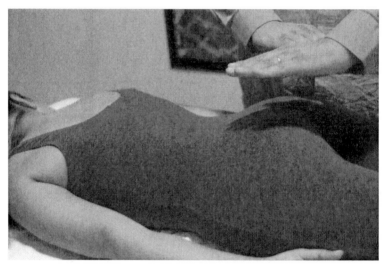

DISTANT HANDS ON THE FIRST CHAKRA
(GLUTEOUS)

TRANSPARENCY ANGELS

Channelling experience with Gaetano Vivo:

Transparent Angels, have come closer to me lately, they came for the first time while I was teaching one of my Reiki three classes, talking to me about transparency. The world needs to be more transparent, it is very important that people look into each others eyes and be sure that whatever comes through is the reality, the transparency of our soul, and nothing else. We are giving help to the people in need; we must do so to help others to understand.

Transparency Angels show me earth, opened like an orange, in one side there are people who are in the light, light workers and energy workers, these are just a few in comparison with people on the other half; on the other side, the heaviest part, people are still in the darkness, we are here to help those people feel more secure, feel more emotional, and open them up to the universal energy which is the beautiful energy that comes from above and which everybody knows.

Transparency is light, it is love, and it is translucency.

The angels are all around us, we do not need to look any closer; they are all here among us…helping us going through life as we perceive it today. We are really changing for the better, light workers need to show us where the light is and how they can achieve it. Light is here, it is within each one of us.

Transparency Angels talk to me about a new earth, a new world where everything will be easier. People need to be more transparent, talking with transparency and more easily.

It seems like, something has to happen to us before we wake up spiritually, if someone dies, or we have an accident, only then is there a wake up call to look around us at angels and spiritual beings. They are here now and forever, wake up, wake up.

You do not want to live in the darkness anymore, it is time now to wake up and smell the flowers, see the stars, look at the sun, get emotional for a sunset or a dawn. Not many people have heard about the transparency angels, they are guided by Archangel Michael and Archangel Metatron

Transparent: like water, like air, like the smoke of candles, like wings.

Transparent like beautiful angel wings.

BIBLIOGRAPHY

1. Baginski, Bodo, and Shalila Sharamon. <u>Reiki: Universal Life Energy.</u> Mendocino, CA.: LifeRhythm Press, 1988, p. 29.

2. Rand, William Lee. <u>The Healing Touch: First and Second Degree Manual</u>. Southfield, MI: Vision Publications, 1998, pp. I-18 --I-20.

3. Stein, Diane. <u>Essential Reiki: A Complete Guide to an Ancient Healing Art</u>. Freedom, CA: The Crossing Press, 1995, p. 9.

4. Mitchell, Karyn. <u>Reiki: A Torch in Daylight</u>. St. Charles, IL: Mind Rivers Publications, 1994, p. 10.

5. Takata, Hawayo. <u>The History of Reiki as Told by Mrs. Takata</u>. Southfield, MI: The Center for Reiki Training, 1979, audiotape and transcript.

6. Graham, Vera. "Mrs. Takata Opens Minds to Reiki." <u>The San Mateo Times.</u> 17 May 1975.

GAETANO VIVO

Reiki Master Teacher Gaetano Vivo has treated and attuned more than 1000 people into the Art of Reiki since 1996.

A Reiki Master of the Usui/Tibetan system, a Karuna Reiki Master with William Rand, and certified Angel Therapist and Medium with Doreen Virtue PhD. Vivo is founder of the Reiki Vivo International School, (formerly the Reiki Wellness Center) with offices in Naples, Milan, London, New York and Gran Canaria.

Prior to starting his Reiki practice in 1995, Vivo founded and operated the Gaetano Vivo Metaphysical Centre in London, England, (1993-1997) to offer workshops, classes, lectures and services, such as psychic and tarot readings as well as books, crystals, art, and music to an international clientele interested in spiritual development, personal enrichment, and furthering their metaphysical knowledge base.

Vivo's path to Reiki as a practitioner began like many others. In June 1995, while visiting London's Body Mind and Soul Expo to look for new ideas for his Metaphysical Centre, he met a Reiki Master who invited him to experience 10 minutes of Reiki. It was the first time he had heard the word Reiki. The 10-minute treatment was extraordinary and, ultimately, life-altering; he signed up for a Reiki I class offered the following weekend and became a level I Reiki practitioner shortly after. Vivo began giving treatments to his staff at the Metaphysical Centre and to himself. That summer while on holiday in Arizona, he became Reiki II. He returned to England committed to devoting his life to healing through Reiki.

In 1996 Dr Vivo became a Reiki Master.

In his lectures all over the world, Dr Vivo talks about the pure energy Love of Reiki, demonstrating his work and clearing blockages and chakras from people randomly taken in the audience.

He gives messages to people with the help of the angels and spirit guides, caressing people's aura, to further enhance pure love for oneself and others.

Vivo uses a variety of healing modalities in addition to and in conjunction with Reiki, including Vibrational Psychic Surgery, going energetically inside the body and clear all the energy centers from blockages. Crystals Therapy, laying of crystals on the body of the client to enhance healing abilities, Karuna Reiki Treatments, toning symbols in the aura of the client in a mantra manner.

Vivo holds a doctorate in English Literature and History from the Oriental University in Naples, Italy. He is an ordained minister, a member of the Complementary Medical Association of Great Britain, the International Council of Holistic Therapies, the International Association of Reiki Professionals, a Registered Professional Member of the International Massage Association, and a member of the Noetic Association of America.

Vivo counts members of the English aristocracy, noted business executives, artists, and entertainment professionals among his clientele. His work has been featured in print publications in England as well as on English and Italian television and radio.

In 2006, Reiki Vivo will introduce, *Beauty from the Inside Out*, a special Reiki program, with emphasis on the seven main chakras (energy centers), to be offered in spas. Vivo is also developing a program incorporating multiple healing modalities including color, sound, aromatherapy, and crystal therapy.

He has published two books on Reiki in Italy "Risveglia il tuo Cuore col Reiki" July 2001, and "La poesia del Reiki" Nov 2004. He has also released meditation Cds in English, Italian, and Spanish, and a KarunaVivo Cd, to enhance relaxation and healing in the world.